STRON MIND
STRONGER BODY
STRONGER LIFE

Build the confidence and resilience
to meet life's challenges head on

GAVIN MEENAN

RƎTHINK PRESS

First published in Great Britain in 2020
by Rethink Press (www.rethinkpress.com)

© Copyright Gavin Meenan

Cover image © Shutterstock | Arak Rattanawijittakorn

Contents

Introduction

As you're reading this book, you're probably looking for answers. I mean, just look at the title – *Stronger Mind, Stronger Body, Stronger Life*. It must have piqued your curiosity, so this wakeup call may be exactly what you need.

Many of us don't know what it means to be good men anymore. Our notion of what constitutes a 'real man' has vanished over time. In the past, it was clear-cut. A real man was someone who fought in wars, provided for his family, worked in a hard manual job, never showed emotion...

Tremendous leaps forward in society have created great progress, but as a direct result, we men have lost ownership of the things that once defined us. Our identity has become complicated and the changes are difficult to adapt to. Without obvious, easy ways of defining ourselves, we seek to prove our manhood through exaggerated expression and overindulgence. We damage ourselves with porn, alcohol and other toxic substances. We weaken our bodies through lack of use (or overuse and abuse of performance-enhancing drugs), and fail to do the things that would make us truly fulfilled.

But the truth is that none of this matters. The ideals that we feel we have to live by are irrelevant. They were made by society, not us. We need to throw out our preconceived notions of what an alpha male or a real man looks like.

I'd like you to consider these questions:

- What do you want from life?

- How do you want to feel?

- Who do you want to spend your time with?

- What do you want to look like?

- Who do you want to be?

If the answers aren't so clear for you, don't worry – just give it time. The little voice inside your head that speaks nothing but the truth is probably hoarse from years of trying to drown out the bullshit, but if you listen closely, you can hear it.

I don't have all the answers, and I'm not pretending to. But that doesn't mean I can't help you, the same way I've been helping myself for years now. That's who this book is for – guys like young Gavin, barely out of his teens, unaware of how little he knows about life and how to achieve his dreams.

When I reflect on my path, I can see that it's like the one so many others have walked throughout time. I'm calling this the path of the strong – because, even though I don't want you to go around kicking people's arses, we are still *all* warriors, and there are more kinds of strength than just physical.

In my definition, a warrior is not someone who wields a sword, wears armour or raids rival settlements with his band of brothers. A warrior is not someone who steamrollers his way through life, crushing any and everyone who stands in his way. A warrior is not someone who seeks out conflict at the expense of all those around him.

The life of a modern man is different to what it was in the past. While our ancestors fought and killed to protect their loved ones, the need to fight has all but disappeared nowadays. But if a warrior doesn't need to fight, then why do we need to become one?

Well, think about it. There's a reason we all love a good hero (and not just the kind we see on the big screen). Think of people you find inspiring. It could be Gandhi,

Mother Teresa, Rosa Parks, Martin Luther King or even Jesus. Their stories inspire so many because they exemplify what it means to be a true warrior. They might not use swords or guns, but they still fight for what matters to them.

We too must fight for what matters to us. Instead of taking his place on the battlefield, a modern man can pursue the mission of building a business, raising a family, writing a book, or mentoring disadvantaged youngsters.

Your meaning is found in your mission. And your mission is unique to you. No matter the journey you're on, becoming a modern warrior is the key to success. By following the path of the strong, you can become the man you need to be to make your dreams come true. That's what this book aims to do: lay out the path of the strong for you to follow, so you can become who you're meant to be.

The modern man has two main weapons at his disposal:

- A strong mind: he takes control of his mind, manages his base impulses and directs his focus towards his chosen mission

- A strong body: he hardens his body into a weapon, one that serves him well on the path

Mastering your mind and body will help you to achieve your goals in all areas of life: your diet, your finances, your relationships and more.

But Gavin, if this is all true, why doesn't every man know about it?

There's an obvious reason why the majority of men don't live like this. It's become easier than ever to make a living in jobs we barely tolerate, working with people we don't like. It's easier than ever to eat poor-quality food, get no exercise and numb our negative feelings with porn, alcohol or other drugs, sinking deeper and deeper into a rut.

Plenty of people have this kind of life. But when they reach the end – when they're lying on their deathbeds – what do they feel? Are they happy they frittered away their lives? Or do they regret the choices they made? Do they wish they could go back and do it all over again?

I've no doubt it's the latter, and I aim to save you from that fate.

To make this book as valuable as possible to you, I've broken it into two parts:

1. The Strong Mind

2. The Strong Body

By focusing on each key area, we'll simplify the path of the strong – the journey we all must go on to become who we're meant to be.

I've written this book with young men in mind – people who are just starting out on their journeys to better health and fitness. But that doesn't mean it's not useful if you're in your thirties, forties or fifties; in fact, it's relevant for older men as well. It's never too late to change and start living a better life. The information in this book has the potential to change your life if you put it into practice. It's had an incredible impact on me – and I know it can do the same for you.

Today is the first day of the rest of your life. Stick with my path, and you'll look back on this as the point where everything changed for the better. Or you'll look back on it as the chance for change that escaped you. The choice is yours. I can guarantee you that it'll make you a better man, but only you can take that first step.

The path awaits you – if you're willing to walk it.

PART ONE
THE STRONG MIND

'Victorious warriors win first and then
go to war, while defeated warriors go
to war first and then seek to win.'
— Sun Tzu, *The Art of War*

1
The Principles of a Strong Mind

Battles are won and lost in the mind before they're ever fought in the physical world. Your success in achieving a new goal (no matter what that may be) is based on your mindset. With the right mindset, there isn't much you can't do.

Let's take one of the simplest examples, and it's one that I'm familiar with from my work: trying to lose weight. In my career, I've worked with hundreds of people who are struggling with the process of losing weight. Sometimes, there are specific reasons why they're struggling (eg one client had a clinical vitamin B12 deficiency, which impacted their energy levels significantly). At other times, their struggles are harder to pin down, but can usually be traced back to a negative mindset. The way they view the world has a great effect on how they interact with it.

Losing weight is a *process*. If we've got a lot of weight to lose, it'll take time; and when something takes a long time, it's more likely that we'll slip up along the way. Sometimes, we'll miss a single workout, then let that snowball into two weeks away from the gym. In that time off, we ignore our meal planning as well – after all, what's the point in healthy eating if we aren't working out? Or maybe we miss one workout, then immediately schedule it for the next day. The difference is clear. The first example shows a negative mindset, and the second a positive one.

Someone with a negative mindset laments that they lack time. A positive mindset gets up early or stays up late to make time. A negative mindset will say they have no willpower to change their lifestyle. A positive mindset asks an expert for the best strategies for maximising willpower and building new habits or researches the topic in their own time. I'm sure you don't need me to tell you which mindset sees better results.

It's the same for any goal, whatever it may be: the actual work you put in might only account for 20–30% of your success. The rest is down to your mindset.

It's your primary weapon; without a good understanding of it, success will be impossible. In this section of the book, we'll be talking about a range of topics that'll teach you how to master your mind. Specifically:

- The mental shifts you'll need to gain mastery over your mind. These will show you the world in a different light, helping you to learn more mental control as quickly as possible.

- The core practice of mental strength (emotional mastery) and how you can start building this skill today.

- Motivation – what it is, how to harness it and how to 'hack' your motivation for endless energy and drive.

- What you need to know about discipline and willpower – how to build them, control them and use them to maximum effect in your life.

- How to form the habits you want and break the ones you don't.

Mastering your mind is the most important thing you'll ever do. Without that mastery, you'll struggle to achieve even 10% of what you're capable of. But with it, you're likely to find the process of achieving your goals easier, quicker and more enjoyable than anything you've ever done.

To get things started, let's look at what I consider to be the six core principles of the strong mind:

1. The strong man understands that vision is everything. Without a clear picture of where he's going, he has nothing to strive for.

2. The strong man understands that life happens in the here and now. He doesn't distract himself with frivolous pursuits or thoughts of the future and past – he faces life head on.

3. The strong man understands that how he begins does not determine where he ends. He is capable of doing anything he wishes, so long as he is willing to pay the price.

4. The strong man knows that 1% improvements compound. Over time, he can become ten times the man he was by committing to the process of consistent, positive change.

5. The strong man understands that stress is good, as it provides him with the opportunity to grow.

6. The strong man understands that today's decisions shape his future. He treats every decision he makes with the respect it deserves.

We'll dissect each of these principles in more detail throughout this chapter.

Principle 1: Mission is everything

Throughout this book, I'll reference the idea of the modern man's mission. To me, a man's mission is composed of all the things he's called on to do as a man. It's his reason for walking the path of the strong in the first place; the challenges that demand he rises to meet them without flinching away.

In broad terms, we all have the same mission – to become the best we can be, build the best lives we can and achieve our dreams. But while our general mission might be the same, the road to get there will be different for every one of us, paved with the goals we'll achieve along the way, such as:

- Owning a business

- Starting a family

- Competing in a strongman competition

- Buying a house

- Travelling to dozens of countries

- Learning a new language

- Leaving a lasting impact on the world

The list is endless.

The strong man masters his mind and body so he can fulfil his mission, but it's only by engaging with his heart that he figures out how to do so. Your goals are personal to you and I can't tell you which are the right ones. Ultimately, the truth lies within you. And when you find that truth, you'll use it as your guide to navigating the outside world.

You can use these exercises to help you figure out the path to your mission.

EXERCISE 1: WHAT MOVES YOU?

The easiest way to start figuring out your path is to consider the things that fill you with emotion. Emotions can be positive or negative, depending on the circumstances, and both can provide valuable clues to what your mission is.

First, think of the things that make you angry. What has the power to make you see red, even when you know you shouldn't react? I'm not talking about minor annoyances like getting cut up in traffic or having to deal with rude clients at work; I'm talking about the stuff that makes you angry because it's unjust. For example, when you see that the rainforests are being cut down at a faster rate than ever before, do you care? Or is it just background noise? When you hear of yet another business taking its operations overseas to reduce costs, does it fill you with anger? Or do you shrug it off as more of the same?

If you view something as unjust, there's a good chance you hold the opposite to be fair or right (ie it's something you value). And clues like that can give you a useful nudge towards figuring out what your mission is.

Note that there's a difference between being pissed off about something and actually doing something to make things better. It's easy to lose yourself to anger and waste your days ranting about everything that makes the world as fucked up as it is, but just being angry about something isn't enough. Anger can be channelled as an engine for action; it can inspire you to do work that needs to be done. But spending a day being angry doesn't mean you've spent a day doing anything worthwhile. The action that follows anger is a vital step.

On the other hand, what things make you happy? Is there anything you do that causes the hours to fly by? What do you do purely for the enjoyment you get out of it? What do you enjoy doing for the process and not the results? I'm not talking about process-based vices like drinking, gambling or watching porn. Think more along the lines of coaching your child's sports team, helping a friend overcome a challenging personal problem or closing deals at work. The things you enjoy are likely the same things you value – and more often than not, those values will point you to the goals to focus on.

EXERCISE 2: REFLECT ON YOUR LIFE

For this exercise, you don't need much: a pen, paper and some time. How much time? Depends, but the more you have, the better. The longer you spend on this, the deeper you'll be able to dig into the truth of your mission.

I want you to think back over your life and reflect on the times you felt happiest and the most engaged with everything around you. How were your days spent during those times? What kind of work did you do? What were you working towards?

When you've finished that, think of the times where you were most unhappy; when life seemed to weigh a thousand tons and nothing you did could snap you out of it. How were you spending your time when you felt at your lowest? What factors contributed to your troubles?

Take some time to really work through these questions – the answers you give (and the obvious differences between them) will prove useful in showing what you need to focus on. For instance, many people would say that they were happiest in their careers when they had control over their schedules and successes; when they were creating real value for their clients; when they were in great shape; when they could devote their time to creative work; when they were learning a language for their next trip abroad; when they could spend lots of time with their loved ones. On the other hand, the stuff they did when they were at their lowest provides insight on how to avoid feeling that way in the future.

If you know that you were at your worst when you were drinking four nights a week and constantly hunting for another one-night stand, maybe you should limit your drinking and focus on developing high-quality relationships. Similarly, if you hated working a job where you had to constantly deal with negativity, then you know you should steer your path clear of that kind of work.

Think carefully about the best and worst times of your life. These memories have important lessons to teach you – you just have to be open to learning them.

EXERCISE 3: YOUR PERFECT DAY

When imagining your perfect day, chart out what you'd like your life to look like from the moment you wake up to the moment your head hits the pillow at night. To help frame this exercise, you can use prompts like:

- What time do you wake up?
- Alarm or no alarm?
- Where are you?
- Who are you with?
- What do you do when you wake up? Morning routine, or freedom of choice?
- Do you have breakfast? What do you have to eat?
- Do you meditate? Exercise? Read? Journal?
- What do you do once you're ready to start the day?
- What do you do for work/impact/fulfilment?
- Do you have a job? Work as a freelancer? Own a business?
- Do you have to work or are you living off passive income?
- When do you take your first break?

- What do you do? Go for lunch? Alone? With someone?
- What do you do after lunch?
- What time do you finish working for the day?
- What do you do then? What's the plan for the evening?
- Do you spend time with friends? Family? Partner?
- Do you spend time volunteering/contributing?
- Do you have a pet or pets?
- Do you have a family?

The point of this exercise is to create a full picture of what an ideal day would look like for you. It's not a fantasy about waking up at noon, lounging on a beach hammock all day, then hitting the clubs that night. Your goal is to determine what a normal day would look like for you if everything in your life was perfect.

Take time to consider the various aspects of this exercise. To do it properly, you'll have to find answers to a lot of big questions (like whether you want a family, your desired career path etc). If you get stuck, Google is your friend – this exercise is popular enough that you're only ever a few clicks away from dozens of examples to give you inspiration.

Vision is everything. Unless you know why you're walking the path, you'll struggle to continue in the face of adversity. The smallest problems will seem like massive mountains, impossible to overcome. But when you get in touch with what drives you, you will harness your true potential. You'll instantly gain access to the power lying deep within you. And with this at your disposal, you'll be able to keep going, no matter what life throws your way.

Principle 2: Be present

While you may think that time travel is a modern fascination (see cinematic masterpieces such as *Back to the Future* and *Hot Tub Time Machine*), our desire to transcend time is nothing new. Our ancestors relied on the wisdom of witch doctors, druids and shamans to reveal the mysteries of fate. The Vikings, Romans and ancient Israelites relied on omens and signs to predict the outcome of a battle before it was ever fought. Belief in reincarnation and past lives is fundamental to many Eastern religions.

Time travel is more than an easy way for writers to justify a weak plot; it's something we do every day, just not in the way we may imagine. Meditation and mindfulness practice have never been as popular as they are right now, and there's good reason for that: as a society, we have a new habit of time-travelling instead of living in the present moment. We look back, ahead and anywhere but at what's right in front of us.

The course of life is like a river. Awareness of what's behind us is useful, but not crucial; we'll never swim in that part of the river again. And being aware of what's coming up is only useful as long as we don't get lost in the rapids right in front of us. People find benefit in meditation or other mindfulness practices because they force us to put aside the bullshit and just be. That's the real magic of meditation – it makes us do what we need to do as humans – but modern society has erased our memory of living our life in the moment rather than travelling through time.

Once our eyes are open, we see time-travelling behaviour everywhere we look. It's in the lad in the gym who's scrolling on his phone for five minutes between sets; it's in a public conversation between social-media-obsessed friends or partners; and most of all, it's in all of us. Notice how often you allow your mind to wander over the past or future, neither of which you can do a damn thing about right now. Because here's the fundamental truth to life:

The only moment you will ever experience is here and now.

The future won't happen until it happens, and when it's here, it won't be the future – it will be now. But if you've conditioned yourself to never be present in the moment, you'll miss it; you'll be waiting for the next future, thinking things will be different when it finally arrives.

The power of full presence can't be understated. Think back to the times you felt most alive – for example, the last personal best you set in the gym. What did that feel like? Tough, I bet. Now compare that to your typical warm-up sets. How much do you remember about those? Odds are, not much. Unless something happens to bring you back to the present moment, your mind wanders.

Think of all the moments you've missed through your time-travelling. How many meaningful conversations have you allowed to slip by unnoticed? How much beauty has gone unseen? I'm not knocking the value of reflection or the power of goal-setting. Time-travelling is useful. It allows you to learn from your past and plan for the future. But doing it excessively is terrible for both you and everyone you're close to.

Being able to stay in the present moment is a powerful skill to develop. With it, you'll be able to work harder and be more effective in the gym. You'll be able to fully engage with the people you love. You'll be able to experience every moment as intensely as if it were your best.

I'll talk more about meditation later on in the book, but for now, I'd recommend you incorporate a basic practice into your day-to-day life. Look up a guided meditation on YouTube, download an app (Headspace and Calm are both great) or just sit and be aware.

The only moment you can experience is here and now. When your mind is mired in the past or drifting towards the future, you're time-travelling. That's a useful thing to do, but don't get caught up in your head and miss life unfolding right in front of you.

Principle 3: The beginning is not the end

It's a sad reality: sometimes, life's going to knock you on your arse. And if you're trying to get in better shape, build better relationships, start a new business or achieve a personal goal, it's going to knock you so hard, you'll have to go to accident and emergency for the bruising.

All of us face hardship. Some live easier lives than others, but we're all hit by it at some point. And when we want to become more than we are right now, we're *choosing* to take on more hardship than we have to.

Everything has a price, especially your desires. The bigger your desire, the bigger the price to be paid. It's unlikely that you're aiming to become a professional athlete, run a billion-dollar company or star in a block-buster movie. Maybe you are – and if that's the case, more power to you – but most people want different things in life. They want to have a strong, good-looking body. They want to do work they enjoy. They want to play an instrument, travel the world, run a marathon...

It doesn't matter what your desires look like, so long as you acknowledge that you have them. But whatever you want to achieve, you have to remember these two rules:

1. There's always a price to be paid

2. Bigger goals require bigger sacrifices

While your goals might not be massive in absolute terms, you can bet your arse there's a price to be paid. That price could be money, time, health, relationships – the trade-off depends on what your goal is. Getting stronger for everyday life is easier than pulling an aeroplane in a timed event. Getting a degree is easier than building the next Facebook. Training for a 10 km run is easier than training for a spacewalk. But within reason, you can do anything you want. Sure, you probably won't play in the National Basketball Association if you're only 150 cm tall, but there's a lot more to life than the hyper-success we see on television. You don't need to be the best in the world – you just need to be the best version of you.

The beginning is not the end. Where you start does not determine where you'll end up. I can't guarantee you'll ever win a bodybuilding competition, become a millionaire or perform on stage in front of a cheering crowd, but you can get better than you are now. And that's all that really matters.

Principle 4: 1% better

When we want to change our lives, we often go hard from the start. We don't ease into our new workout or diet; we fly into it with 100% intensity, dedicating ourselves entirely to that new vision of who we are. And sometimes this works, but most of the time, it doesn't. That's why so many fail at their diets, fail at their workouts, fail to quit smoking, fail, fail, fail, fail, fail...

Motivation is great while we have it, but the decisions we make while high on it are never as appealing in the cold light of day. Our motivation gets used up over time. And when that happens, we stop trying to change. We go back to the way things were and get further away from living the life we desire for ourselves.

If you can relate to this, just know you're not alone. Practically everyone has done it – yes, even me. But over the years, I've learned that it doesn't work. Sometimes, we've got to be realistic. Instead of going all-out from day one, I've found it useful (both in my own life and in coaching) to start small. Don't try to change your life overnight; focus on getting 1% better.

Maybe 1% sounds small. Hardly worth the time it would take to make it happen. Better to burn yourself out reaching for the stars than settle for a nearby hill, right? But if you improve by just 1% every day, you will make amazing progress in a year – an unbelievable amount.

Here's the equation for anyone who cares: $1.01^{365} = 37.78$, which in words means that getting 1% better every day (1.01 multiplied by itself 365 times) means being thirty-seven times better at the end of one year.

Contrast the all-out approach of burnout to someone who focuses on making 1% better decisions every day. Instead of ploughing into the gym six days a week from the start, maybe they go for a twenty-minute walk after their dinner. Rather than radically overhauling their diet overnight, they focus on little things like not taking sugar in their tea, giving up drinking calorie-heavy drinks or eating more vegetables with their dinner.

These are small changes. At first, they won't seem like they're making a difference, particularly when you compare yourself to the guy who hits the gym every day and starves himself when he gets home, but they're *sustainable*. Three months in, the guy who charged in head-first has burned out and quit, while you've graduated to strength training twice a week, eating a relatively balanced diet and getting enough sleep every night. You're in a position to make better choices as you continue to get 1% better every day.

Don't doubt the power of 1% improvements. Every day, you can choose to get 1% better or 1% worse. And even if losing 1% of your progress doesn't seem like much, remember that no choice is made in a vacuum. Your choices stack and fall like dominoes. The decisions you make today influence the ones you make tomorrow.

It's good to have big goals, but the choices you make today matter even more. Make sure that what you're planning can *actually* be done consistently, or you'll find yourself back at square one. Improve just 1% every day, and in a year, you won't believe how far you've come. Start small and let tomorrow take care of itself.

Principle 5: Becoming antifragile

Author Nassim Nicholas Taleb is famous for writing about economics, but his work has applications for self-improvement as well. In his book *Antifragile: Things that gain from disorder,*[1] he lays out a formula for building strength. He described systems as falling into one of three categories:

1. Fragile

2. Robust

3. Antifragile

Fragile systems are like fine china: they look pretty, but they break easily. They respond poorly to stress

---

1   N N Taleb (2013) *Antifragile: Things that gain from disorder.* London: Penguin.

and need to be protected from anything that could harm them.

Robust systems are a little tougher. Think of them like the plastic cups you let a kid drink out of. They can take all sorts of abuse – you can throw them around, drop them on the floor, put hot liquids in them, but over time, they still wear down. *It's still possible to do damage to them.*

Stress is of no use to a robust system. At best, it does nothing, and at worst, it causes irreparable damage. In this sense, fragile and robust systems are similar. They'll both fall apart; it's just a matter of when.

An antifragile system doesn't just tolerate stress; it *thrives* on it. It needs it. Without stress, an antifragile system may as well be a fragile one, because it'll never look any different.

Your body is antifragile. You get better when you push yourself to improve beyond what you're capable of, and becoming stronger is the easiest way to become antifragile. By pushing yourself through physical discomfort, you ensure your mind becomes stronger too. You'll be better able to cope with life's stresses. Your comfort zone will expand until the things that once frightened you won't look as intimidating anymore.

Your body is antifragile – and so is your mind. To become better, you have to go through pain. Stress will make

you stronger in the end. You just have to be willing to
see it.

Principle 6: Work today, benefit tomorrow

Many young men don't give the future much thought.
Sure, they'll pay lip service to building a better career,
a stronger body, healthier relationships with the people around them, but when it comes down to it, they
prioritise short-term gains over long-term success.

This is a huge issue, and it's one that I've personally
struggled with. For my teen years and early twenties,
I was obsessed with enjoying myself in the moment,
and my choices reflected this. Binge drinking. Watching
porn. Chasing shallow relationships. The things I did
brought pleasure in the short term, but in the long run?
They held me back from becoming the man I knew I
could be.

I believe that if we truly understood the consequences
of our actions, we'd make better decisions than we do.
One way I like to do this is by looking at my life path
as a marathon instead of a sprint. What do I need to do
to make sure I get to the finish line without a sprained
ankle?

Instead of worrying what the effects of your actions
will be in six months, ask yourself, 'Where will I be in

ten years if I keep doing this?' That's the right way to judge your actions. Small decisions compound over time to govern where you end up. Good decisions will lead you to a positive destination and bad ones will lead you astray.

This concept of marginal gains is explored in greater detail by Jeff Olson in *The Slight Edge*.[2] The book's fundamental message is that the things that make a real difference in your life are easy to do and easy not to do. They're small decisions, basic disciplines. For example:

- Skipping a workout today won't set you back in the grand scheme of things, but skipping every workout for the next ten years will.

- Going to bed angry once won't ruin your marriage. Doing it every week for years will spell the end of your relationship.

- Wasting money on a frivolous purchase today doesn't matter, but a habit of poor financial discipline will ruin you in the long term.

Habits are a crucial part of what makes us who we are. They can see our vision for the future through to becoming a reality when we choose them well. But if we neglect to do the things we know we need to do,

---

2   J Olson (2013) *The Slight Edge: Turning simple disciplines into massive success and happiness.* Lancaster: Gazelle.

that destination will get further and further away until it's nothing but a speck on the horizon.

Time will pass, regardless of the choices you make. So in ten years' time, where will you be if you continue on your current path? Where do you *want* to be? The things you do today will decide how your life turns out ten years from now, just as everything you are right now is a result of the choices you made when you were younger. Leaving aside sudden tragedy or genuine randomness, you have direct input into how your life turns out. Whether things work out well for you is largely in your control.

The modern man understands this. Like stones in a wall, each day stacks on top of the one before it. A poorly laid stone will affect those that come after. A well-laid one will be the foundation for future success. The choice is yours.

This doesn't mean you can never take the time to enjoy life. If you want to drink, despite knowing that you'll feel it the next morning, go for it. Fun is fun and your life is your own – I'm not here to dictate how you should live. But ten years is a long time and it's important to commit to doing the right thing for most of it. The actions of today shape the results of tomorrow, and the actions you choose are entirely up to you. Never lose sight of the bigger picture. You're not here to win today and fade away tomorrow; you're here to build a better life for yourself.

Three exercises to reflect on

There are three exercises that many people could benefit from to help set them up to live better lives in the years to come. I'd like to close this chapter by outlining these three exercises briefly, and then I'll share the case study of a man who turned his professional, fitness and personal life around by adhering to the six principles we've just covered.

EXERCISE: FORGIVE THOSE WHO HAVE HURT YOU

In life, we're going to encounter people who piss us off. Family members, friends, colleagues, strangers. Whatever the cause, people are going to rub us up the wrong way. And it's easy to hold on to that feeling. As humans, we carry grudges around for years. Long after the annoyance has passed, we dwell on it. We wonder what we ever did to deserve this treatment, why it had to be us who felt that way, and contemplate ways to get revenge.

I've been there. I've been treated poorly by people and looked forward to the day I could get them back for it. Sometimes, that feeling pushed me through the bad times. But holding on to negative emotions isn't good for anyone's wellbeing.

That's why forgiving the people who have wronged you isn't just for their benefit – every bit of baggage you carry weighs you down and makes things harder than they need to be. And on the path of the strong, every gram of additional strain will only slow you down.

Save your focus for the people who matter. Not your childhood bullies; not the ex who cheated on you; not the boss who skipped over you for a promotion. Forget that bullshit. Distance yourself from the people who bring you down – don't spend time with them, interact with them or even think about them.

Forgive. If not for the other person's benefit, then for your own. Don't carry around the weight of past hurts when you don't need to.

EXERCISE: ACCEPT THAT DISAPPOINTMENT AND FAILURE ARE PART OF THE PROCESS

Failure hurts. It's the biggest thing that holds men back from becoming stronger. They're afraid of looking stupid and can't bear to see that their inflated self-image isn't real.

But failure and disappointment aren't signs you should stop. They're a crucial part of the process.

Without figuring out what doesn't work, you have little chance of succeeding in the end. Unless you stumble on the winning formula your first time out, failure is unavoidable. What is avoidable is viewing that failure as failing.

The bigger the failure, the more you can learn from it. Pain gives way to growth if you allow it to do so. That's what separates it from pointless suffering.

Detach yourself from the bullshit stories you're likely to tell yourself. You're better than them so don't fall for your own lies. Take whatever genuine lessons you can from your experiences, then use them to do better moving forward.

The biggest life lessons I've learned have come from my worst mistakes. You'll probably find the same is true for you.

EXERCISE: BECOME BETTER

The lives we live are largely a product of our choices. Poor choices beget a poor life. Good decisions lead us to better outcomes, so the results we get are a product of who we are.

People who engage in healthy practices (working out regularly, eating well, getting enough sleep) enjoy the outcomes of better fitness, health and energy levels. People who cultivate the habits of being honest, open and vulnerable with loved ones have better relationships. And those who manage their spending have more money than those who can't even spell 'budget', let alone plan one out.

But blaming others for the situation we've put ourselves in is easy. Victims can't be expected to succeed – it's someone else's fault, so what can we do? This mentality is disempowering. If someone else is in charge of our results, we're subject to their whims and nothing we do matters. And life isn't like this. The way we live our lives is – mostly – up to us, so we all need to build better habits.

STRONGER MIND, STRONGER BODY, STRONGER LIFE

Take responsibility for yourself. Stop blaming others and figure out what you can do to improve your situation. You can be your own worst enemy – if you choose to be. But you can also be your own best friend. The choice is yours. And I think it's a pretty easy one.

CASE STUDY: ANDY'S MARRIAGE WOES

Andy was the kind of man that other men envied. From the outside, he looked like he had it all: a great job that gave him a solid six-figure income, a huge house, a fancy car, four holidays a year to five-star resorts, a loving wife and adoring family. But on the inside, things weren't so rosy.

As a travelling tech consultant, Andy was constantly on the go – 24/7 availability, weeks on the road and overseas trips at the drop of a hat. That's what his job really required of him. And with a career like this, Andy (understandably) didn't have much time left over to look after his health.

Years of poor eating and little exercise were starting to take their toll on him. All those expensive dinners and drinks with clients had left him with more padding than he would have liked. Besides that, he was also starting to feel run-down (his diet wasn't exactly conducive to vim and vigour). He had a clear vision of where he wanted to be, both physically and mentally. All in all, he was ready to make a change.

That's where I came into the picture. Andy approached me, figuring that I was the guy to help him get a handle on his situation. Over the course of twelve weeks, I worked with Andy to create a bulletproof exercise and diet plan he could adhere to, no matter what his crazy schedule required of him. I pushed him to stick with the plan, the small improvements to get 1% better each day, keeping him in the present and accountable via regular email check-ins. And his results were impressive. At the end of this first three-month block, he was starting to look and feel like a warrior (not someone who had neglected his physique for ten+ years).

My work with Andy had been nearly 100% online, but to cap off our twelve weeks together, he decided to pay a visit to Sligo for a final meeting. He wanted to get clear on his strategy moving forward – and of course, I was more than happy to help him with this.

We had spoken a few times via Skype over our months working together, so I already had a good feel for the type of man Andy was. He was someone I admired, to be honest – it looked like everything was going well for him, and I was happy that I had been able to help him get another area of his life in order.

After a productive session in the gym, Andy and I popped down to the local to relax with a few drinks and chew the fat. And it's over these drinks that Andy confided in me that all was not well with him.

Years of travelling and sacrificing himself for the job had hurt more than just his fitness. Andy's relationship with his children and his wife had deteriorated. He told me that pretty much all of their interactions were negative these days.

Family was always important to Andy. He had met his wife in college, and had instantly known she was 'the one'. Providing for her (and the children that soon followed) was a priority for him. Giving her and his kids freedom was all he really cared about.

And in this day and age, the fastest path to freedom is paved in cash. So Andy focused on his career, giving up his time, energy and life to secure financial comfort for his loved ones.

That's why he spent all those years on the road, putting in long hours until he was one of the most valuable, sought-after people in his industry.

That's why his health and fitness had taken a back seat for so long.

He told me he was tired of sacrificing his life for a job and was ready to make some serious adjustments. He had already talked to his superiors about taking his current role remote. No more wasting time sitting around in fancy offices, clocking up a day rate. His end goal – his vision – was to spend at least three weeks per month working from home so he would have more time with his family.

Now in his mid-forties, Andy felt he had earned this respite. But he was worried that things with his wife were doomed to never improve, despite his best efforts. I empathised with Andy. As someone who had chosen to give up so much to ensure his family could live a good life, he felt terrible about the way things had turned out. He was wondering if he had wasted his life up to now in pursuit of a goal that was forever out of reach. The situation looked bleak. But it's human nature to magnify our own problems. We're too close to them to truly understand how to solve them.

Andy loved his wife. He loved his kids. He wanted to make this work. That was half the battle, I told him. But what about his wife?

Andy went quiet. I could tell he was reflecting back on the past twenty years, truly trying to think of an answer to my question. When he looked back at me, there were tears in his eyes.

I told him that the fact his wife exhibited frustration at him was a sign she still cared about him. If she had felt that their problems couldn't be solved, she probably wouldn't have wasted her energy engaging with him. If she was angry towards him, she knew he could do better. He could be a more active part of the family. And if Andy was committed to making things work, if he was willing to pay the price, he could. No doubt in my mind. The specifics of how he'd do it didn't matter too much, I told him. The lifestyle changes he was choosing to make to spend more time with his family would speak far more loudly than words ever could. In the end, all that his wife needed was to know that Andy loved her and would be there for her more moving forward.

Earlier that day, we had agreed to work together for another twelve-week block, helping Andy further cement the good habits he had built during our previous stint. As we parted ways, I reminded Andy that I'd be in touch the following weekend and I'd expect him to keep me updated about what was going on.

True to his word, Andy kept me in the loop with regular updates on his workouts. His progress was impressive for anyone, but was amazing given everything else he had going on. After three weeks of regular accountability, I broached the topic of his marriage at the end of one of my update requests. The reply soon came in: things were looking up.

Today, Andy and his wife have strengthened their relationship even further. The old hurts of past neglect have been washed away. Andy now spends more time than ever with his family, freed up to do so by his new career.

All it took to kick start their recovery was a simple gesture on Andy's part. But without having been vulnerable and open enough to admit things weren't good (without being antifragile), he never would have had the courage to confront the problem head on.

I'm lucky to have met a man like Andy. And I'm incredibly grateful I was able to play a part in helping him build a better relationship with his family.

2
Managing Your Emotional State

Learning to manage your emotional state effectively is the single biggest thing you can do to improve your ability to handle stress, overcome setbacks and stay on the path to achieving your goals. But some men would lead you to believe that emotions are bad: extra fuel for the fire at best and a meaningless distraction at worst. And there's some truth to that. Taking action to pursue your goals will sometimes mean that you have to do things when you don't feel like doing them.

I believe it's important to distinguish between motivation and emotion. We'll talk more about motivation in the next chapter (including some strategies you can use to boost yours and make the process of attaining your goals much easier), so for now, let's address emotion.

It's no secret that your mental state at any given moment can influence how you feel about putting in the work to achieve your goals. On days where you're happy and upbeat, it's fun to sit down and grind through your tasks in pursuit of something bigger. But on those days where your mind is foggy and you can't see a reason to go on – how easy is it to act then? We've all been there before, so I'm sure you know the answer.

Mental reframing

Many of the most effective forms of psychotherapy focus on giving you the skills you need to better process your emotions. That's because learning to do this is a huge part of building a stable foundation of mental fortitude, an asset in any endeavour. Hands down, the single most impactful skill I've ever come across is known as mental reframing (or recontextualisation, depending on who you talk to). It's simple, but when you put it into practice, it's incredibly powerful.

What is this technique? In a few words, it's changing your perspective on a situation or event to change how you feel about it.

As humans, we all have our own unique set of cognitive biases, distortions and filters we use to interpret the world around us. These filters are formed consciously and unconsciously over the course of our lives. The people who raise us, the media we consume, the things that happen to us all play a part in shaping how we see things. Of course, there's nothing to say that your particular set of filters is accurate. In fact, they could well be what's holding you back from reaching the next level (whatever that means to you).

Few things in life are good or bad for their own sake; we decide what they mean to us. For instance, say you're involved in a car accident and, miraculously, walk away unscathed. The other driver, however, is fatally injured. That event, in and of itself, is a tragedy, but the long-term impact of it is up to you.

You could take this horrible situation and use it as a catalyst for improvement, campaigning for road safety and legislative change to prevent that kind of thing from happening again. You could speak to young drivers about the dangers of speeding, or drink-driving, or driving while under the influence of illegal substances. You could equally take this tragic event as evidence that life has no real meaning and fall into a spiral of distraction and self-medication with alcohol and other drugs to take your mind off reality. You could refuse to ever get behind the wheel of a car again, and instead rely on other people to drive you around.

That single event could lead you to many different places – and it's safe to say that some of them are more empowering than others. The underlying reality doesn't change. That other driver is still dead and you are still alive. This situation doesn't have any inherent meaning; it's up to you to decide what it means.

Let's take another example. Back when I was in college, I frequently found it hard to sit down and work on assignments in good time before they were due. A lot of them ended up being last-minute jobs when I let the fear of an impending deadline spur me into action. Looking back now, I can see that the meaning I gave to the situation affected how I felt about it. I saw these assignments as pointless bullshit – stuff that had to be done to tick the boxes and get a piece of paper that would allow me to start doing what I wanted to do, which was helping people as a personal trainer. In my eyes, this work was just an obstacle.

But what if I had chosen to see those same assignments in a different light? What if I'd viewed them as a necessary stepping stone towards achieving my overall goal of becoming a personal trainer? What if I'd viewed the act of sitting down and commencing work as an exercise in discipline – a skill that would be of tremendous help to me in the future when I was chasing even bigger dreams?

The work was the same either way, but the meaning I attached to it could have made *all the difference*. Rather than putting off what needed to be done until the last minute, I could have used it as an opportunity for personal growth. And it's the same no matter what we're talking about.

- Sticking to your guns and getting to the gym – even when you're tired after a long day at the office – could be a painful obligation you don't feel like completing, or a chance to build a great habit that you can rely on again in the future.

- Breaking up with your girlfriend after finding out she was cheating on you could be the worst thing that ever happened to you, sending you into a downward spiral that takes months to recover from. Or it could be an opportunity to work on yourself, become a better potential partner to attract higher quality people into your life, and a lucky break (because it is better to find out that she's a cheat now rather than later).

- Losing your job could be a huge setback. Or it could be the opportunity to find a job that you enjoy more and the chance at a better life.

It's important to note that there's a difference between what's true and what's empowering. When you break up with your girlfriend, there's no way to objectively know if it's a good or bad thing. Maybe you could have built a happy life together, or you could have broken up for something else a month later. But without any hard data to go on, why assume the worst? Why choose to believe it's horrible when there's no evidence to back that up?

When tragedy strikes you down, why make that heavy burden impossible to bear by piling your own perceptual baggage on top? Why not seek to learn the most empowering lessons you can from that event? And when you struggle to remain consistent with your diet and exercise routine, why take that as a sign that you can never change? Why not look at your overall approach, or maybe even view your struggle as part of the process?

We can't always control what happens to us, but we can control how we interpret these events. The events that befall us are nothing but words on a page in the book of our lives; *we* determine what comes next.

Learning to reframe everything that happens to you is the single most important mental skill you can develop. With this weapon in his arsenal, the strong man will be able to better manage his emotional state (which will help him commit more easily to the process of achieving his goals). But please note that this is not an instant fix; it's a skill you have to develop. Don't be disheartened if you find it difficult at first. If you've been stuck in a negative headspace for a long time, it'll take some time to get out of those old ways of thinking. But believe me, it's worth it.

This skill is also great for working through events in your past. Depending on the kind of life you've lived up to this point, it's quite possible you're carrying emotional baggage with you, left over from some long-ago event. The interesting thing is that how you feel about this event can change in an instant.

For example, imagine that your parents separated when you were young. You don't remember much about it, but you know that one night, your mother took you away from the family home and you both moved in with her sister for a time. You soon found a home of your own again, but your father never reappeared; you grew up without ever knowing him.

In this situation, it's possible that you'd harbour a lot of resentment towards your mother. You could feel that she deprived you of something important and you pin the blame for most of your problems squarely on her. Well, what if it transpired that your father had been abusive towards her, and the night she left, she had taken you away for your own safety?

As soon as you learn this new information, your perspective changes. You start to see your entire childhood in a different light. Your mother stops being the person responsible for you not having had a father growing up, and you finally see her as the loving, protecting parent she has always been. In mere moments, years of unhappy childhood memories could become something different.

The core skill of recontextualisation will allow you to move past any events that are holding you back from becoming the man you're meant to be. If you're ready to make serious change in your life, I recommend you complete the three exercises I'm going to share now. It's important to work through them in order. Like any other skill, you have to practise reframing a lot before you'll be able to do it on command. It won't be easy, but it will be worth it. That much I can guarantee.

EXERCISE: REFRAME MINOR ANNOYANCES

The first exercise I'd like you to work through is pretty easy. All you need to complete it is some time to yourself. Feel free to work through it on paper if you feel that helps, but I find it just as effective to talk myself through the process out loud.

Reflect on the past week and think of a few times where something has negatively impacted on your mental state. This could be something as simple as a minor argument with your partner, a tough conversation at work or someone taking a parking space you had your eye on. Whatever it is, bring it to mind.

Then ask yourself, 'What positive lesson can I learn from this experience?' or 'What empowering meaning can I draw from this experience?' In either case, your goal is the same – to reframe how you think about that minor annoyance.

Let's take the example of an argument with your partner. Depending on the subject matter, you might find it difficult to take anything positive away from it, but bear with me!

You could view it in a negative light and see it as another example of how your partner is always nagging you; how they love to argue; how your relationship isn't going that well right now. Or you could take some useful meaning from it. You could, for instance, see that conflict as an indication that you need to get better at communicating. You might see it as an opportunity to develop your patience and understanding. You might even see it as a good thing – if you can resolve the conflict in a productive manner, you and your partner will grow even closer together. And you want your relationship to get stronger, don't you?

That's a simple example, but an effective one. And all of your other minor annoyances could be reframed in this manner too.

- A conflict with a colleague at work could be a chance to develop the skill of asserting yourself and staying cool under pressure
- Someone cutting you up in traffic could be a chance to practise safe driving and demonstrate how aware you are as a driver
- Stubbing your toe on the kitchen cabinet could be a (painful) reminder to be more careful when you're walking around the house

Do some of those sound silly to you? If so, that's fair, but it doesn't diminish their usefulness.

I've often found that little negative experiences compound over the course of a day. While none of them are that significant in isolation, they can stack up to have a serious impact on your mood when taken together. By learning to reframe these little annoyances as they happen, you'll be able to prevent them from having an effect on your mental state moving forward. This, in turn, will help you to see more of your experiences as positive throughout the day; being unburdened by the niggling negatives will free you up to see the goodness all around you. Over time, you'll be able to instantly reframe minor annoyances. They'll have zero impact on you; in fact, they'll be a good thing as they'll give you a chance to reinforce the valuable reframing skills you've developed up to this point.

After you've tried this exercise, you'll be ready to move on to...

EXERCISE: REFRAME THE PAIN OF PROCESS

Once you've built the skill of reframing little annoyances, you'll be able to start looking at routine activities in a different light. Pretty much any goal worth chasing is going to require you to follow a process to achieve it. For example:

- Getting in great shape requires you to stick with a solid diet and training routine for months at a time
- Earning a qualification requires you to study, complete assignments on time and pass exams
- Building a good relationship with your family will require you to spend time with them and develop better communication skills

And so on. But we don't always feel like doing the things we know we need to do. No matter how attractive the end result is to us, staying excited and engaging in the routine, day in, day out for long periods of time, is emotionally taxing. Just as we often see minor annoyances in a negative light, we also see routine actions as little more than a bothersome obligation. But we can reframe them.

Take the skill of reframing little annoyances that you learned in the previous exercise and put it to use again here. Think of the actions you have to engage in on a regular basis. To keep things simple, let's stick with the goal of physical transformation as an example, but feel free to apply this same thinking to any actions of your choosing.

Let's say you've figured out that transforming physically is going to require you to: ·

· Hit the gym four days a week following an intelligently designed workout routine

· Eat 3,000 calories a day, balancing your diet appropriately

· Sleep at least eight hours per night

Those actions seem pretty simple on the surface, but when we dig a little deeper, it's easy to see how things could get more complicated. For instance, it's all well and good to say you'll hit the gym four days a week, but maybe the thought of driving to the gym after a long day at work, completing your workout, taking a shower, driving home, then preparing a meal seems like more hassle than it's worth. If you're in a negative headspace, it's easy to see all of these parts of the process as mere drudgery. But you can actively shape your perceptions to succeed, taking an empowering view of what you do.

Let's look at two opposing perspectives you could take when thinking about all of the little actions that make up the process of getting into better shape. For the sake of simplicity, I've labelled these two viewpoints as disempowering and empowering respectively.

Disempowering:

- Driving to the gym is shit. Waste of time. Why is there so much traffic? Why didn't I go earlier? Why don't I just go tomorrow?
- I'm too tired to hit this workout properly. I'll make up for it the next day.
- I can't get comfortable in this shower. The water isn't hot enough.
- I'm too tired to cook something complicated. I'll just grab a pizza on the way home and call it a day.

Empowering:

- The drive to the gym is my chance to get in the zone. I'll put on some good music and visualise the session ahead. I'm confident I'm going to hit some new personal records tonight, and I'm all about personal growth, so that's a big deal for me.
- I've had a long day, so I'm looking forward to the chance to unwind by letting off some steam with these weights.
- The shower and drive home will give me some time to reflect on my workout and consider what I can do to improve next time.
- Cooking my dinner when I get in gives me the chance to engage in some mindful activity before I shut down for the night. It'll be nice to practise

being in the present rather than always looking for a distraction.

The actions are the same in both cases; all that changes is how you see them. Having a disempowering perspective makes the process too painful to be worth it. If you do manage to push through those negative feelings and put in the work anyway, you'll end up wasting much more energy than you need to. By learning to reframe the actions you have to consistently take to achieve your goals, you'll be able to spare your willpower for more important things. Rather than having to force yourself to go through the motions, you'll instead enjoy doing so. And when you enjoy the process of chasing your goals, it goes without saying that you'll have an easier time sticking to the path.

I find that this exercise is a good one to work through on paper because a written list of the reasons why the process is enjoyable (and not just a hard slog) will be a useful reference for those days when you just can't get motivated to work. Once you've got a good handle on reframing the process, you'll be better able to tackle this third exercise.

EXERCISE: REFRAME YOUR WORST MOMENTS

Reflect on your life and make a list of the three worst things that have ever happened to you. This could be the loss of a loved one to cancer, incidents of brutal bullying, the end of a meaningful relationship, an injury... anything that has had a serious negative impact on you.

Once you've got that list, I want you to do something difficult. Ask yourself, 'What empowering lessons can I take from this event?'

This won't be easy. In fact, you might wonder how on earth you're supposed to learn anything from the tragic loss of a loved one, a freak accident or anything horrible you were put through. I understand your confusion, but push through. Let those initial negative feelings swell up and fade, then focus on what you came here to do.

If it helps, distance yourself from the situation a bit and think of it this way. If you knew someone who had gone through this situation, what empowering meaning do you think they could take from it?

Your answers will be personal. Some of them might provoke a gut reaction. You might even resist your answers, thinking that they're too stupid/shallow to make a difference. Persist. Be objective. Find the empowering meaning you can draw from the situation.

When all is said and done, the strong man's first – and most important – battle is with his own mind. If the baggage of years gone by weighs heavily upon you, you'll have a difficult time raising your weapons for the battles that lie ahead. It's up to you to figure out what you can learn from the things that happen to you. Life hands you an experience; you determine what to make of it.

These exercises are simple, but they are far from easy (particularly the last one). Over the course of years, many of us have been conditioned to look for the worst in any situation. Whether we're afraid of things going sour, quick to jump on the negative, or just pessimistic in general, the result is the same: preoccupied with the thorns, we fail to see the beauty of the rose before us.

Remember, it's up to you to decide what anything means. Nothing has an inherent meaning; you decide what is good or bad based on your perceptual filters. And if those filters aren't serving you? Take on this challenge and master the skill of mental reframing. You'll benefit – today, tomorrow and ten years from now.

Now that we've talked about emotion, let's tackle motivation.

3
Hacking Your Motivation

We've all had days where we feel unstoppable. We fly through work, crush a hard workout, have great interactions with people and generally bounce around, loving life. On the other hand, we've also experienced the opposite. We drag ourselves from obligation to obligation, counting down the seconds until the painful day finally draws to a close.

There are a lot of factors that contribute to how we feel on any given day. It can be something as simple as how much sleep we got the night before (that's actually a huge factor), if we've eaten well or if we're under stress. And obviously, when we feel bad, our motivation to do certain things takes a nosedive. That's why sleep, diet and exercise are the first casualties when we're under pressure with work or studies.

What if it was possible to hack your motivation so you felt like doing these things anyway? I'm here to tell you it *is* possible. It's not a guaranteed fix, but it's certainly better than nothing. And the day you need it, this technique could make all the difference.

Pre-commitment

To explain how this works, let's consider an example. You're taking a pleasant stroll down a country road. It's the middle of June. The midday sun above is casting a warm glow over the landscape and a cool breeze makes the heat tolerable. You feel at peace – you think nothing could ruin this moment.

You see a stream in the distance. A large oak tree sits on the bank, tempting you to come closer and enjoy the shade. You hop over the nearest wall and start to cut across the field, already looking forward to basking in the comfort that awaits. You're so caught up in your fantasy that you fail to remember the warning sign you spotted a few minutes back.

You're snapped back to reality by the distinctive huffing of an irate bull. In this moment, do you think you need much motivation to get your arse in gear and jump back over that wall as quickly as you can?

An obvious criticism of this analogy is that it's an extreme life-or-death case. Maybe it's not perfectly applicable to something smaller, like you skipping out on your workouts or failing to stay on your diet. Fair point – the immediate pain of a charging bull is a lot scarier than feeling a little unhappy with yourself for not sticking to your plans, so let's look at another example.

Cast your mind back to when you were studying for exams or trying to complete some important assignment. If you were anything like 95% of college students, you had problems with procrastination. It was all fun and games early on in the year – you had plenty of time to catch up on what you were doing. But as the deadline drew nearer, you couldn't escape the feeling that you were in trouble. All of a sudden, you wanted to get your work done; you knew that there would be serious consequences looming if you didn't.

In this situation, were you worrying about how to get motivated? When it came down to the wire, no. While you may have been lamenting all the time you wasted in the preceding weeks, the consequences of missing that deadline were motivation enough to get you going.

The common thread between both of these scenarios – the charging bull and a looming college deadline – is the immediate consequence of failing to act. In your quest to build a better life for yourself, how can you use this lesson for your own benefit? Simple: by pre-committing to something and finding an accountability partner.

Pre-commitment is where you agree ahead of time to do something. Your to-do list or schedule lays out what you plan to do on a particular day, but these are weak examples of pre-commitment in action as the consequences of failing to cross off all your tasks are minimal. But if you get a little more creative in how you use this tool, you can unlock its true power. For example, you could:

- Give €500 to a friend to hold for three months. If you're good and hit all your workouts, you'll get the full amount back. But every time you miss a gym session for some bullshit reason, they get to spend €25 for themselves. Or €50. Whatever hurts.

- Sign up to enter an event, for example a 5 km or a 10 km run, with friends. You don't want to be shown up in front of them, so you'll have extra reason to train on the days when you don't feel like it.

Money is an easy tool to use as you probably have some of it to hand, but aren't inclined to throw it away. Attaching a financial penalty to your failure to complete certain actions is an effective motivator. When the alarm goes off at 6.30am and you're about to roll over to go back to sleep, you might think twice if your gym partner will be waiting outside for you at 7, or you might not. But if you know that you'll have to pay them €25 for the privilege of those extra few minutes, suddenly your bed won't seem quite as comfortable.

The key with using pre-commitment effectively is to hold yourself accountable. In theory, you could do this alone, but in reality, the outside pressure of having to report to someone else is great for keeping you on track. This is particularly true if you can find someone who will call you on your bullshit. Skipping a workout when you can't stop throwing up is smart; giving it a miss because you 'feel a little tired' isn't. Having someone who accepts the former but not the latter is invaluable.

Good accountability partners are hard to find. This is because the people closest to you are often willing to cut you more slack than you deserve. This special treatment is born of love, but can ultimately hold you back from becoming who you want to be.

Working with a coach can be great for accountability. One of the main benefits of hiring a personal trainer or online coach is that you're forced to pre-commit (by paying them upfront), and then check in with them regularly (ie be accountable to them). Consider seeking out a coach for your area of interest. This can be huge in keeping you on track, so don't neglect it.

You may be thinking that pre-commitment and account-ability seem pretty negative. While they're not inher-ently this way, the truth is that we fear loss more than we value gain. If there's no consequence of failing to do something, we have less incentive to actually do it. An opportunity to gain €100 is less appealing than acting to save €100 we already have (for most people, at least).

But positive rewards can also be a powerful motivator. We'll touch on this in more detail in a later chapter on building habits, but for now, let's just say this: the value you attach to your actions will influence how motivated you are to complete them. The question is, what do you value? And what influences your perception of value? Fundamentally, it comes down to two forces that drive everything you do.

CASE STUDY: REWARD AND ACCOUNTABILITY

When I first met Marcus, I didn't know what to make of him. I had known Marcus's older brother Patrick at college, and he was the life of the party. No matter what our plans were for a night out, Patrick was up for a laugh. He was the kind of guy no one had a bad word to say about; you couldn't help but like him.

I hadn't seen much of Patrick since graduating from college over ten years previously. He had moved to Australia shortly after getting his degree, secured a client-facing sales role – no surprise, knowing the man he was – and started making tons of money. But despite our different paths, I always made the effort to meet him when he came back around Christmas time. And it was during one of those December evenings down the local that he brought up the topic of his brother.

Patrick had kept his easy-going nature as he matured, but when he talked about Marcus, there was something in his tone that made me sit up and pay attention. Gone were the laughs and jokes. It was clear there was more going on here than I was privy to.

Patrick didn't see a lot of his brother, but he had kept in touch with him since moving away. Apparently, life was proving tougher than Marcus had expected. He was staying up late, getting up late and generally not living up to his potential. Patrick had heard that I was good at getting people out of their ruts, so he wanted me to do the same with Marcus.

Marcus was still living locally, so it would be no trouble to take him on as a client. Patrick was delighted and we made plans for Marcus to come by the gym I was working at the following afternoon.

When Marcus arrived the next day, I was taken aback. I had been expecting someone like Patrick – all smiles and laughter. But the young man before me was the exact opposite. It was like there was a dark cloud hanging over him.

I went over to see what the story was with my new protégé. 'How's it going – Marcus, is it?' I said, sticking out my hand.

His eyes shot up to meet mine, then darted away as he limply returned my handshake and mumbled a greeting.

On the outside, I was positive and professional. But on the inside, I knew I would have my work cut out to help him.

Our first session was an easy one. I put him through his paces (he wasn't in bad shape), but my main goal was to get a sense of who he was as a person. There was something about him that reminded me of myself at that age.

When life feels like a noose around your neck, one way to get a little breathing room is to focus on improving in one small area. Before long, those small improvements spill over into other areas of your life too. For Marcus, I guessed that there wasn't really much in his life he was improving. So the first thing we could do was help him see improvements in his strength and body composition. But I knew that getting him interested in this project was going to take some creative thinking on my part. Fortunately, with a little help from Patrick, I soon created a solid plan of action.

Marcus was absolutely crazy about cars. He had passed his driving test on the first attempt a few days after turning eighteen, and one of the few things he still enjoyed doing was taking his car for a drive around the local area. Since he didn't have much money, he was limited in his choice of vehicle, but like any other car nut, he had a shopping list as long as his arm of all the upgrades he wanted to make.

When Marcus came back two days later for his second session, I was ready to go. Before we began the workout, I took him to one side and explained the deal. For the next sixteen weeks, he would come to the gym four days a week to train with me. My hourly rate at the time was €50 per session. As a favour to Patrick, I had said I'd take half that, but Patrick had insisted on paying the full amount on Marcus's behalf. Rather than keeping my friend on the hook for paying the full amount directly to me, I had come up with a better plan.

Marcus would show up for our first session with a balance of €0. Every time he put in what I considered to be his best effort, he would 'earn' €25 for the session, and I would take the other €25. Every time he missed a session or showed up without putting in any effort, he would basically 'lose' €50 of Patrick's money. At the end of the sixteen weeks, Marcus stood to gain a maximum of €1,600 – a huge amount of money to any unemployed teenager. But when I subtly reminded him that €1,600 would go a long way towards upgrading his car, he was sold.

Over the next sixteen weeks, Marcus showed up like clockwork for each of our sessions. Four days a week, he pushed the pace on every exercise, training like a man possessed. I suppose it was no surprise – he was getting paid to do so, and it would cost his brother money if he didn't perform.

At the end of the sixteen weeks, Marcus was a new man. His physique had improved substantially, going from average to defined, and more importantly, when he walked into the gym for our final session, he looked me in the eye, grinned and said, 'Let's do this.' Just like Patrick and I had hoped, the gradual improvements he had made in this small area had enabled him to start making positive changes in all aspects of his life.

The last I heard, Marcus had completed a four-year civil engineering degree and was working with a big construction firm. I feel grateful to have had the opportunity to help that young man come out of his shell and start living a better life.

The two forces that drive everything we do

No matter how complicated we try to make it, there are really only two forces that drive everything we do:

1. Our desire to seek pleasure

2. Our desire to avoid pain

It's simple, but it's true. Pretty much anything we've ever done (or failed to do) can be explained through this paradigm.

Don't go to the gym consistently? You're avoiding the pain of working out and indulging in the pleasure of whatever else you're doing (sitting around, watching TV or Netflix etc). Can't motivate yourself to study for exams? You're avoiding the pain of staying in and hitting the books rather than going out with your friends. Been putting off a visit to the dentist to get that toothache checked? You're avoiding the pain of paying over money, facing your fear (if you have one) and having to deal with reality, instead hoping it will go away on its own. But when you really get into it, what causes certain behaviours/actions to be linked with pleasure and others to be linked to pain?

We're getting into murky waters here. Questions of psychology rarely have a straightforward answer. Two people who engage in the same behaviour (eg going to the gym consistently) could have different reasons for doing so. One could enjoy the positive mental-health benefits associated with their workouts and the other could be using the gym to destroy themselves after a rough breakup. The end result is the same (both work out), but their reasons for doing so differ.

I can't tell you why you do or don't do certain things. But I can show you how to change what you link pain to and what you link pleasure to. By getting this kind of leverage, you'll be able to reduce the amount of effort it takes to act. You'll run away from pain and towards pleasure anyway, so why not control these things?

I've found this exercise to be helpful:

EXERCISE: CREATING STRONG PAIN AND PLEASURE LINKS

In the previous chapter, we discussed reframing your habitual actions as things that you look forward to doing. We'll be doing the same thing here again, but rather than just looking at the small actions you have to take, we'll be analysing the big-picture goals you're chasing too.

It's natural for your motivation levels to be low when you have no real reason to do something. It's your body's way of preserving precious energy. If something isn't meaningful, why waste your time trying to attain it? Better to save that effort for the things that really matter, which, from a survival perspective, are the basics like food, shelter and reproducing. But if you've got big goals beyond just surviving, you'll need to run through this exercise to change what your body and brain attach significance to.

Our brains have a tendency to place a priority on short-term pleasure over long-term success. That's why a sugar high is more attractive than eating a healthy meal. It's why porn is more attractive than the struggle of building a meaningful long-term relationship. It's why getting drunk is more enjoyable than doing the hard work of managing our emotional state without relying on substances. But the short-term pleasure we get sets us up for more problems in the future.

To reframe how we view things, we need to get clear on how much they're costing us in the long run and minimise the pleasure they're giving us right now. For instance, let's say you have a habit of skipping out on your meal plan and eating shitty food on a regular basis. Here's how your brain would typically view this action:

Avoid pain	Gain pleasure
Short term:	Short term:
• Avoid having to put in effort to cook something healthy	• Tasty food right now
	• Feels good not to have to put in effort
• Avoid wasting your time on a diet that might not even work for you	• Save time to spend on scrolling on your phone or watching Netflix
Long term:	Long term:
• ???	• ???

You don't really think about the long-term consequences of your actions, because if you did, you'd see that you're making the wrong choice.

To get around this, let's take an objective viewpoint. Pretend you're sitting with a friend who's engaging in the same problematic behaviour. Because you're eager to help them change their lives and eliminate this issue, you get them to think about the impact of their behaviour. With no prompting, they come up with exactly the same answers as to how their behaviour brings them pleasure and avoids pain.

This is your starting point. But to enact real change, you have to go further. For the next step, you're going to flip the script. To get a full picture of why the negative behaviour of eating unhealthy fast food has to change, don't ask how it's helping you gain pleasure and avoid pain; instead, ask how it's costing you pleasure and bringing you pain.

Gain pain	Avoid pleasure
Short term: • Indigestion, inflammation and negative impact on your mood • Reduced recovery between workouts • Less motivation to do other things	Short term: • Lose out on the satisfaction of sticking to your plans • Don't feel energetic (like you would if you ate well)
Long term: • No progress towards your fitness goals • Bad health • Less attractive to potential partners • No energy to pursue big goals • No self-confidence • No discipline being built • Risk of diabetes, heart disease, other serious problems	Long term: • Harder to attract great partner, so you miss out on this • Miss out on being energetic and good health • Miss out on having the energy to pursue and achieve your goals • Miss out on the satisfaction of improving your physique • Miss out on building discipline which you can use elsewhere

Not looking so attractive now, is it? The real benefits of this approach are seen in how they help you reframe the long-term consequences of your actions – the minor benefit of eating something tasty right now pales in comparison to the long-term damage your bad habits are causing.

Once you've got crystal-clear on the need to change, you need to figure out what the correct action to take is. In this case, it could be to stick to your meal plan and only indulge in scheduled cheat meals once a week for the next six months. When you take the time to sit down and analyse your behaviour in this way, you'll quickly be able to see how certain things are holding you back from becoming the man you want to be. Then you'll have a much easier time making better decisions in the future.

To apply this exercise to your life, start by making a list of your bad habits. Here's a list of common ones:

- Chronic procrastination
- Not being consistent with your workouts and diet
- Being too loose with your money
- Drinking too often
- Gambling
- Watching porn
- Spending too much time on social media

Whatever's causing you problems, look at it objectively and figure out what pain and pleasure you associate with it. Get clear on how you might be contributing to it, and how you might correct it going forward.

This isn't a cure-all, particularly if you have a genuine addiction. Remember: there's never an advantage to taking on these problems alone. If you need to, seek professional help. The skills you'll learn in this book will help, but there's no substitute for working with an expert, particularly if you want to get a handle on your problems in a hurry. This exercise simply aims to help you overcome one huge stumbling block many people struggle with in their quest for self-improvement: not being able to delay gratification.

CASE STUDY: JACK'S FEAR

As a personal trainer, I worked with many people who sought to change their bodies for many different reasons. Some people had grown up in environments that nudged them towards making unhealthy decisions. Some people had been pushed down the road by a single bad decision they made in their youth – that first cigarette or hard drink had spiralled out of control, leaving them in desperate need of help. And others had no real story to tell. Their health was average. Their bodies were average. But inside, they felt trapped. Their true potential remained locked up by a body too weak to express who they truly were. That's how it was for Jack, although I didn't think it at first.

On the surface, Jack seemed like many of my other clients. A few years into college, he was a little underweight, but not in bad shape. He was reasonably consistent with his training, not great with his diet, paid a bit of attention to recovery. I didn't envision us having too many problems working together.

I worked with Jack to create a routine that he could follow in his college gym. After that, we touched on diet. My goal wasn't to make him neurotic about food choices or to stop him having a few drinks on a night out, just to temper it a bit. He had no questions or concerns about the plan I'd laid out, so I was happy enough to see how he got on. I told him I expected regular check-ins via email, which he was happy to agree to.

When the weekend rolled around, he sent in his first update. And something felt off to me. He had failed to complete one of his sessions for the week. Not the biggest deal in the world, I reasoned – three out of four wasn't bad. He'd probably just had a late night out and couldn't muster up the energy to go. Not ideal, but not concerning. But when he missed two sessions the next week and didn't complete any the following week, I knew something was wrong.

I pushed Jack to see what was going on. Why was he missing his sessions? He said that the gym was too crowded when he was going first thing in the morning and the equipment he needed was always in use by the time he arrived. Something I had seen many of my college-age clients benefit from was working out late in the evening, when the gyms were quiet. I suggested that to Jack and he was on board with the idea, saying he'd give it a try.

Another week went by. When his next update email came in, I was taken aback to see he'd failed to complete any sessions for the second week in a row. I pushed for an answer. What was going on? And the answer surprised me.

Jack told me he was afraid to go out by night. During his first year in college, he had been mugged while walking back to his accommodation alone after a night on the town. He'd survived the incident without anything worse than a black eye, an empty wallet and a bruised ego... or so he'd thought. But when it came time to head off on another night out, Jack said he was too busy. He had exams coming up; had to be up early the next morning; he was tired... His friends accepted his excuses the first few times, but when they kept hearing the same responses to their invitations, they stopped bothering to invite him.

When I suggested that he work out last thing at night instead of first thing in the morning, he had agreed in principle. But deep down, Jack had known he wouldn't try. The idea of walking to and from the gym by himself at that time was too scary to confront.

It was clear to me that Jack's problem wasn't motivation, or confusion about the plan. No, his challenge was fear. Jack needed to talk to someone. And by the sounds of it, he wasn't comfortable talking to any of his college friends about it. So I decided that we'd arrange a call and help him overcome this challenge.

After some general chitchat, we got around to the main purpose of the call – helping him overcome the fear that was keeping him indoors at night. In his own words, Jack told me he knew this was about more than just being able to use the gym by night. His social life had stagnated, which was making his mental state much worse. And the fact that he was letting this fear dominate him meant his confidence was at an all-time low.

First off, we talked through some basic safety tips – don't walk home alone after a night out; don't get too drunk; keep to well-lit pathways (no dodgy shortcuts); move quickly; attract minimal attention. After that, we turned to the issue at hand. How could he get past this event that was holding him back?

I reminded Jack that, scary as the mugging was, it was something that was unlikely to happen again, assuming he wasn't a total moron and took basic precautions. After that, I gave him a quick tip that I've found useful in my own life: exposure reduces fear. The more you do something that scares you and see that nothing bad happens, the more you'll come to realise that the fear is just in your head. It's not reflective of reality.

Weeks passed. Each week, I received a little update from Jack. He followed the process I had laid out. First, he got comfortable with being just outside his safe zone at night, then somewhere else on campus. Then he got familiar with the path that scared him so much, walking it with a friend. And finally, the day came where Jack walked that path alone.

Despite how insignificant it may have appeared on the outside, it was a huge win for Jack. And the newfound confidence that came with beating his fear spilled over into other areas of his life too. After another few weeks, Jack was excitedly telling me he was finally going out on the town with his friends again. They'd been glad to see him back – he was the life of the party when he got going.

With this mental issue taken care of, Jack was able to restart our twelve-week coaching package. He went on to make great progress in our time together, smashing personal bests with consistent action and a newfound dedication to the process. Most importantly, Jack developed into a stronger, more confident man as a result of overcoming his fear. The event that had victimised him had been reframed as a challenge – just one page in the book of his life, not the defining end of his story.

Delayed gratification

Our beliefs as to what will bring us pleasure and what will cause us pain are tied to our perception of time. As humans, we're all predisposed towards 'temporal discounting'.

In simple terms, temporal discounting is seen in how we place far greater value on things that are available to us right now, and much less value on things which will be available to us in the future. Think of it this way – if I offered you €100 today or €110 a month from now, which would you take? Most people would take the €100 today, rationalising that they would rather have the money than wait for a little more in the future. And sometimes, that's the right decision – maybe they need money right now, and I just happen to come along at the perfect moment. But in purely financial terms, they'd earn more if they could just wait.

While this sort of thinking has obvious applications to personal finance (if you can save some money over time instead of spending everything you earn, you'll be better off), it's also relevant to anything else you're interested in doing – making a change to your physique; learning a new skill; building a business; whatever. When it comes to improving your health and fitness, results aren't always apparent right away. After enjoying the initial gains you get as a beginner weight-lifter, for example, progress slows down considerably.

If you've been training for any length of time, you're not going to pack muscle on fast – less than half a kilo per month in most cases (assuming you're not getting fat along with it).

When the future reward is small (eg it'll take a year to gain 4.5 kg of muscle) and far off (a year is a long time when you're starting off), you often discount its value. Suddenly, it's hard to justify this investment of time, energy and toil. So you seek ways to bring the reward closer. You think you could be doing 100 different things that are better. You could jump from one program to another, searching for the perfect workout to give you gains faster than ever before. You could take steroids and shortcut the process entirely. You could even quit and find something else to do with yourself.

Bringing this back to pain and pleasure – even if you associate pleasure with the end goal (gaining 4.5 kg of muscle), temporal discounting means the pain you associate with the process of getting there (working out, eating well, getting enough sleep, staying consistent) will be far greater. And when the pain outweighs the pleasure, you're not likely to succeed.

Delayed gratification refers to our ability to put in work now so we can earn rewards in the future. Your ability to delay gratification will significantly impact the quality of your life. Master it, and you'll succeed. Ignore it, and you'll fail.

If you struggle with delaying gratification, there are a number of things you can do.

- You can build your willpower and self-discipline, which will allow you to muscle through and do the things you plan to do, regardless of how you feel.

- You can build good habits. Over time, this will allow you to simply take actions that get you closer to where you want to be, without having to invoke 'willpower' to push through.

- You can change how you feel about activities. Either associate more pleasure with them if they are essential to getting you to your goal, or increase the pain you link to them if they are holding you back. This will get your internal motivation mechanisms onside, spurring you towards the right choices with no extra effort.

Think of these approaches as three parts of one whole. If you truly want to achieve important goals, you'll need to use all three of them. Otherwise, there will come a day when you'll fail to keep the promises you made to yourself. You'll need willpower for the days when you feel terrible and can't see a reason to continue. You'll need habits when your willpower is low. And you'll need natural motivation when your habits can't save you. And when you've mastered these three techniques? Sticking to your plans and doing all that you want to do will be easier than ever before.

With that in mind, let's move on to the next chapter and talk about discipline and willpower.

4
Discipline and Willpower

We all struggle to stick to new things sometimes. It could be a workout, a diet, a hobby, or just an important task we never seem to have time for (not today, cluttered spare room – not today). Whatever the case may be, with enough discipline, willpower and grit, we can do anything. The only thing stopping us is us. So we need to be better, do better, become more than we are right now.

There's a lot of truth to this idea. Exercising willpower is a good thing. It's like a muscle – the more we use it, the stronger it gets. Over time, we'll be able to push ourselves further than we ever thought possible. Here's the tricky thing about willpower, though – the science as to how it really works is unclear.

I just compared willpower to a muscle – a power that we can build up over time and draw on more and more as we develop it. But if we really think about it, there's significant overlap between this idea and building better habits. We'll cover habits in more detail in the next chapter, but for now, think of a habit as something you do without having to exert any willpower. A simple example is brushing your teeth. If you're civilised, you brush your teeth twice a day, and it doesn't take much effort to do so. You probably don't even think about it. The habit of brushing your teeth is deeply ingrained, reinforced by years of repetition and social conditioning. So if you believe that willpower is a muscle you can strengthen over time, is this much different to building a habit?

When you build a habit, you reduce the amount of willpower needed to do something. When you increase your willpower, you can force yourself to do more whenever you need to. Both of these actions have the same end result: you stick to your plans, solidify your routines and eventually reap the rewards.

You need to take care of your willpower by recharging enough (eg sleeping, relaxing and eating well – we'll discuss recovery best practices in more detail later in the book). If you're not taking care of the fundamentals, you won't be able to push yourself to take necessary action. But as the majority of people are walking around in a sleep-deprived, poorly fuelled state, it's no wonder they struggle with staying disciplined.

You also need to avoid holding self-limiting beliefs about the amount of willpower you possess. You have a finite amount of willpower, sure – but the truth is you don't know how much you have. It can run out, but it's unlikely you'll reach this point. You can't continue forever on an empty tank, but in all likelihood, you're not even close to being finished.

Your brain makes up just 2% of your body mass, but consumes 20% of your energy. When you try to push past old limits, self-preservation mechanisms kick in, discouraging you from going any further. This is natural, but that doesn't mean you should give in. Pushing on to do more (in a reasonable manner – I'm not saying injure yourself) is good, because it will give you perspective on what you're really capable of. Chances are that it's much more than you think.

Finally, by exercising willpower on a routine basis, you'll improve the strength of your discipline muscle and the efficiency with which you use it. Things that require a ton of mental energy at first become more bearable, and what was once impossible becomes a challenge for you to overcome.

I'd like to help you out now by sharing three of my favourite methods for building and maintaining will-power. I've found all of these methods to be useful at one time or another, so consider using them yourself. Give them a try and see how you feel. After a few months of regular practice, you're likely to find the results addictive.

Technique #1: Cold showers

The cold shower is, without a doubt, one of the most common self-improvement practices out there. From mental toughness, willpower, discipline to health benefits (some questionable, some real), the list of reasons to hop in the shower and switch the dial to 'cold' is long indeed. But few people do so for one simple reason: cold showers are a bitch.

Seriously, it's one thing to take a nice, cold shower when it's 30 degrees outside or you've just finished an intense training session. It's another thing entirely to strip off first thing in the morning, hop in the shower and stand there as you're pounded by an icy waterfall. The thought of it as I'm sitting here, nice and warm, to write this chapter is enough to make me shiver.

But that's the point. It's not supposed to be comfortable. It's supposed to be hard.

There's no real danger in taking a cold shower. Unless you happen to have a serious heart condition, nothing bad will happen to you – beyond feeling uncomfortable for however long you can stand it. You don't take cold showers because they're magical; you take them because they train you to push forward and take action, even when you know that it's going to be uncomfortable. You never really get used to the shock of cold water hitting you. It gets a bit easier with time, but the physiological feeling is the same every time you step in there. What changes is your ability to handle it mentally.

Pretend that you've decided to take a cold shower every morning for the next two weeks. Here's how that is likely to play out.

The first day you step up, you'll dawdle for a few minutes, wondering if there's even any point to what you're about to do. You'll wonder why you're following the advice you read in some guy's book and tell yourself that a hot shower is better for you anyway. Eventually, you'll get in – for as long as you can bear it. Which won't be long. Maybe you'll cheat a little by just putting your feet in or turning it back to hot after thirty seconds. Either way, you've made progress.

The second day, you'll still be slow to get in – you'll not be keen to repeat the experience you endured twenty-four hours earlier. But you'll remember that you felt pretty good after yesterday's shower; you were able to take action and do something outside your comfort zone. Nothing bad happened – why not do it again?

You'll get in and last a little longer than yesterday. Not a lot, but long enough to call it progress.

The third and fourth day play out similarly. You still delay, but you have a couple of successful days behind you now. You know what you're getting yourself into. It sucks, but at least you're prepared for it. You focus on breathing slowly and deeply while you're in the shower. That helps – the water doesn't feel quite so unbearable when you relax and just let it happen.

By the fifth day, you're not delaying quite as much, and you're staying in the shower for longer. By the ninth day, you're letting the cold water run over your whole body – no more sticking a leg in and calling it a win. By the time day fourteen rolls around, you're getting in with little delay and staying in for the full duration. The sensation of the cold water hitting your skin is still uncomfortable, but you don't feel so stressed out about it anymore. And you feel great once it's over. After this early morning win, you're ready to roll on and have a good day all round.

Cold showers aren't magic, but they help you to develop your willpower. They teach you to push forward in the face of imminent 'pain' (discomfort, really) and enable you to build confidence that you can use again when it matters.

If you're interested in incorporating cold showers into your routine, here's what I recommend:

- Do them first thing in the morning. It's a hell of a lot harder to convince yourself to get in there once your day is rolling – and when you're tired after work or school, you'll probably just put it off until the next day (which is never).

- Set yourself a target time to stay in there – three to five minutes is good. And don't cheat by dipping a toe in and calling that a shower – full body!

- Commit to doing it every day for two weeks or a month. It sounds tough, but by the end, you'll understand why they're so popular.

- If you're finding it tough to acclimatise to the cold water, splash some on your face and body before you jump in. That'll ease the initial shock.

Technique #2: Meditation

Meditation and mindfulness practices work. You may already be familiar with some of their more well-known benefits, such as:

- Stress management

- Reduction in anxiety levels

- Better self-control

- Lower blood pressure

- Better sleep

But did you know meditation is one of the most valuable tools in your willpower-building arsenal?

If you've ever tried to meditate before, you'll know that it's tough. Not because there's any physical challenge to it, but because it's often boring. When you're trying to count your breaths, it's difficult to avoid getting pulled away from the practice by random thoughts. When you're observing everything around you from a detached place of awareness, it's easy to get distracted. Your brain is used to being constantly stimulated. If you need any evidence of this, just think of how often you reach for your phone – at work, at school, at home. At the first sign of boredom, you're immediately searching for something interesting to do.

But this is a huge mistake, particularly if you hope to achieve anything significant in your life. If you're unable to bear the mild discomfort of being bored in the quest to achieve your goals, you're unlikely to succeed. Getting in the gym day after day, hitting the same kinds of workouts and exercises is 'boring'. Staying disciplined with your diet is 'boring'. Even trying to focus on the book you're reading right now is 'boring' – you may be multitasking with a TV on in the background, laptop open in front of you, your phone nearby.

Note that I've enclosed 'boring' in quotation marks. Your perception of how engaging these activities are is down to how conditioned you are to constantly seek something more stimulating.

Think back to the chapter where we talked about time-travelling. The behaviours you've reinforced over months and years are the ones you default to and are the hardest ones for you to change. But if they're holding you back, change is worth it – even if it is a struggle. One of the key things that limits the amount of willpower you can exercise is your ability to push through boredom. And the easiest way you can develop this skill, unlocking more willpower than you ever knew you had? Just sit and deal with it. Focus on one thing (your breath, a thought, your surroundings) to the exclusion of all else. Do this for a few minutes a day at first, gradually building up to ten or twenty minutes as you get better.

The first time you do this, you'll see how hard it is. You're likely to do well for the first two breaths, then you may start to think that you're hungry, wonder what you should eat, wonder how long is left before you've finished and can stand up again. Then you'll remember you're supposed to be focusing on your breathing. You'll curse yourself and get back to it. But before long, your mind will be wandering off somewhere else, only to be pulled back and have the cycle begin all over again.

Here's the secret – this happens to everyone. While you'll learn to focus for longer and longer periods of time the more you practise, you'll never entirely escape distraction. But that's OK. As long as you keep bringing your attention back to the matter at hand, you'll be developing a crucial skill for life. And not only that. As you get better at sitting and focusing on one thing for extended periods of time, you'll be unlocking hidden reserves of willpower you never knew you had. The capacity to co-exist with boredom doesn't just help you endure a quick meditation session that feels like an eternity; it also helps you stick to your goals in the long term too.

Many people like to start out with simple guided meditations. It's easier to stay focused when you have someone to talk you through the process, reminding you to stay on track whenever you get distracted. If you're interested, the Calm and Headspace apps are both great. There are plenty of quick guided meditations on YouTube too; just click around until you find one you like.

Willpower is what compels you to move forward when you don't feel like doing anything. Being able to face boredom over and over again (and coming out victorious) is crucial in developing willpower. Meditation is one tool you can use to cultivate this capacity in yourself. Don't be intimidated or put off by the idea it's too fluffy/trendy to be of benefit. Start small – get an app, find some YouTube videos you like and commit to doing it every day for two weeks or a month. You'll soon see the benefits of this practice emerging in all areas of your life.

Technique #3: Pushing yourself one step further

Here's a technique which is simple, but highly effective (if you put it into practice), with the potential to benefit you tremendously over time. Whether you're studying for an exam, pushing for a few extra reps in the gym or putting the finishing touches to a difficult work project, there comes a time when you want to quit. Whatever the activity in question, your inner dialogue looks something like this: 'I've had enough – I've done plenty. Why keep going? I deserve a break. It's not good to work too hard. Better to save myself for another day.'

I'm not going to say these thoughts are never accurate. Getting enough rest and recovery is important. For instance, you don't get bigger or stronger during your workouts. In fact, working out has the opposite effect: the stress it imposes on your body breaks you down. It's by recovering from the workouts that you get stronger, faster, fitter. So there is a point of diminishing returns where doing more work is detrimental to your progress (not just in the gym – all areas of life). If you've ever experienced burnout, got a migraine from working for too long or been so tired that you could hardly keep your eyes open, then you know what this feels like.

But if we're honest with ourselves, we all usually stop long before this point. We rarely push to the point of true failure in the gym – we stop when we feel tired.

We succumb to the temptation of distraction when we should be working, justifying it as a necessary break. We give in without truly testing our limits.

This is a mistake. To build the ability to go further, you have to go further. Your body and mind adapt to the stress you place on them. If you never go a little further, you won't be able to do it when it really counts.

Willpower is what pushes you to take action when no part of you wants to continue. To strengthen your willpower, you need to get out of your comfort zone. Take on a little more than before. Prove to yourself that you're able to do this.

This helps in two ways:

1. By habitually pushing yourself further than is comfortable, you strengthen those pathways in your brain, making it easier to do the same in the future.

2. By proving to yourself that you're capable of going further, you'll undermine self-limiting beliefs that say you're not capable. This helps you to unlock more of the willpower you already possess.

When you feel like quitting – when you're getting tired, you're not sure if you can do another rep or you're getting too 'bored' to continue – double down and push forward. Chances are you'll surprise yourself with how much further you can go.

Exercise a bit of common sense with this recommendation. Don't cripple yourself. Don't work for sixteen hours straight and end up with a pile of shit that's only fit to be scrapped. But when you first feel that urge to quit, keep going. When it hits you the second time, keep going. Feel free to call it quits the third time round.

Over time, you'll find that you can keep going for longer and longer without needing to tap into your willpower. And when you do need to rely on it, it'll take you further. Get used to pushing yourself one step further. Do this regularly and you'll soon have the willpower levels you desire.

These are the three activities I recommend for building discipline and willpower (I use the terms interchangeably as we don't need to overcomplicate this topic), but there are plenty of other practices you can employ, for example:

- High-intensity workouts, designed to test and build your mental toughness

- Fasting for extended periods of time (twelve to twenty-four hours)

- Learning a new language or creative skill like playing an instrument

- Taking a whole day every week to avoid using the internet/your smartphone

Depending on your situation, you may find some of these are better options for you than others. Regardless of what you end up doing, the basic practices of cold showers, meditation and routinely pushing yourself just a little further will serve you well.

Willpower is a valuable asset. You won't always feel like doing the things you know you need to do. When you're not in the mood, it can be difficult to get going. Having a reserve of willpower to rely on in these scenarios is extremely important. Don't neglect building the skill of getting shit done, regardless of how you feel.

But you can't achieve your goals on willpower alone. Like a muscle, it only has so much energy – eventually, if you keep asking too much of it, it fails. Getting enough sleep, eating well, being judicious in your decision-making – all of these things will help you to conserve willpower for when it's truly needed, but it's important to put other systems in place too. Systems that help you to do what you have to do, even when you don't really have the willpower to push forward. Building solid, effective habits is key, and in the next chapter, we'll talk about this in more detail.

5
Building Great Habits

Your habits will make or break you. Build good ones, and you'll reap the rewards for years to come. But if you waste your time ingraining self-destructive behaviours, you'll put yourself on the fast track to ruin.

A habit is defined as a behaviour you regularly engage in without thinking much about it. And because you don't have to think about doing it, it doesn't take much of an emotional toll, ie it doesn't use up your willpower. This is good because your willpower is finite. You may have more of it than you think, but it's limited. If you have to keep forcing yourself to do things you'd rather not be doing all day long, you're eventually going to drain the well dry.

The science of habit-building is well established. Many authors have written extensively on the subject. Two of my favourites are Charles Duhigg, author of *The Power of Habit*,[1] and James Clear, author of *Atomic Habits*.[2] Both of these authors offer great insights into the practice of building solid habits. If you're interested in learning more about this topic, I recommend checking out their works.

What follows in this chapter is a breakdown of the three biggest ideas I've used personally while building better habits. Put these into practice and you'll be well on your way to mastering this critical domain of self-improvement.

Big idea #1: The habit loop

Charles Duhigg is well known for popularising the habit loop, a key subject of his standout work, *The Power of Habit*. Essentially, it tells us that our habits are triggered by a cue which leads us to do something (a routine task) and subsequently gives us a reward. Simple, but powerful if we understand how to use it.

---

1   C Duhigg (2013) *The Power of Habit: Why we do what we do and how to change*. New York: Random House Books.
2   J Clear (2018) *Atomic Habits: An easy and proven way to build good habits and break bad ones*. New York: Random House Business.

If you're building a good habit, you need a cue to remind you to engage in the behaviour. You also need to get some benefit from completing it. If there's no reward, you'll have little incentive to do it.

When you're wanting to build a daily habit, it can be good to link it to a cue that you already encounter as part of your daily routine. For instance, let's say you want to start meditating every morning. You could simply throw it onto your to-do list and 'get around to it whenever', but if you've ever tried this approach, you'll know it doesn't work. At least not consistently (and consistency is huge when it comes to building habits).

Instead of hoping you remember to do it during the day, tie it to something else you already have to do. Maybe put a note on your bathroom mirror reminding you to meditate. When you use the bathroom in the morning, this cue will remind you to engage in your new behaviour.

If you want to build the habit of working out more often, your cue could be to walk in the door and see your gym bag, packed and ready to go from the night before. If you want to build the habit of getting to bed on time (so you can get up earlier and not feel like a zombie), then your cue could be a specially named alarm set to go off an hour before your target bedtime, reminding you to wind down.

Having a logical link between the cue and behaviour is important, as these things are more powerful when they're in context. It should become apparent pretty quickly if you've chosen a poor cue. If you notice yourself habitually forgetting to complete your new behaviour, there's a good chance you need to pick a better cue. If your cue reminds you of your new behaviour (in that you know you should do it), but you still don't do it, it's possible you need to link a stronger reward to completing it.

Over time, you may start to enjoy the activity for its own sake, eg the buzz of a hard workout or the sense of calm after a meditation session. This will motivate you even further to stick to your habits – a powerful asset in your journey to make this behaviour automatic. But when you're just starting out, it can help to stack the deck in your favour.

I'm not talking about eating two pizzas as a reward for working out for thirty minutes or celebrating your five-day meditation streak with a bottle of Jameson – be smart about this. You could decide you won't watch any TV/Netflix/YouTube videos until you've worked out for the day, or that you can't have your coffee in the morning unless you've meditated first. The point here is to choose a reward that doesn't actively work against whatever outcome your new habit is helping you achieve.

Big idea #2: The two-minute rule

When you're starting to build a habit, it can be tempting to jump in at the deep end. You're eager to make your life better. You're confident that you can succeed this time around – you're finally motivated.

But the decisions you make in a peak state are rarely so exciting in the cold light of day. Suddenly, you wonder if you really have time to meditate every day for twenty minutes or hit the gym five days a week. You reason that you can afford to skip a session here and there, as you can always make it up the next day. I'm sure you know how this story ends: inconsistency, falling off the wagon and a general lack of progress across the board.

We're all susceptible to this. It's human nature to think that we can grit our way through when we need to, and that our current motivation levels will never leave us again. With time and experience, we see these are false beliefs. We can use our willpower to get us through sometimes, but given that we're in the process of building habits so that we won't have to waste willpower, that can be counterproductive.

The best thing to do is to start small. And a useful rule of thumb for doing so is the two-minute rule.

In simple terms, ensure that whatever new behaviour you're trying to turn into a habit takes under two minutes to complete. If you want to start meditating, commit to just two minutes. You can shoot for more on good days (eg ten or twenty minutes), but only commit to two minutes.

You might want to start going to the gym five times a week for a full workout. Great – go for it! But if the shit hits the fan and you don't have an hour to spare, commit to getting in two minutes of exercise. Literally. Get down on the floor and do as many push-ups as you can in two minutes. And if you can't do push-ups, do something else.

The point here isn't that two minutes of meditation will lead you to eternal zen, or that one set of push-ups per day is all you need to get huge. It's to build consistency.

Momentum is powerful, whether it's working for or against you. When you don't have much margin for error (eg if your chosen behaviour is a big one, like working out for forty-five to sixty minutes a day), the possibility of failure is quite high. But if you know your minimum for the day is to hit one set of push-ups? You'll always have time for that.

When the worst comes to pass, you'll be glad you established a two-minute version of your behaviour. Engaging in this stripped-back habit will keep you on track, setting you up to reap the benefits of the habit in the months and years to come.

Big idea #3: It takes time

It seems like only yesterday that every self-help guru was parroting the idea that building a habit takes a mere twenty-one days. In as little as three weeks, you could go from zero to hero, effortlessly flossing your teeth, taking cold showers, hitting the gym five times a week and eating a perfect diet on autopilot.

Yeah. Sadly, it doesn't work like that.

From my own experience, different habits take different lengths of time to become ingrained, depending on their complexity. An easier habit might only take a few weeks to develop, while a trickier one could take up to a year. Most fall somewhere in the middle, taking somewhere around two months to become fully ingrained in your daily routine.

That's a little over sixty days of effort on average to build your chosen habit. Not much time, in the grand scheme of things, but more than most people want to commit to. It's easy to get caught up in a self-improvement craze. In an effort to get to your end goal as fast as possible, you bite off more than you can chew. You try to introduce eight changes into your daily routine at once. And maybe you can stick to it for a week or two, but soon enough, you'll slip up. And when you miss one day, it's easy to justify another. And another. Until eventually, it's been weeks since you gave it a proper try – right back to square one.

Here's the hard truth: changing your life takes time. It's not an overnight deal. It's going to take weeks, months and years of solid effort to get where you want to go.

That's not to say you can't make great progress if you're just starting out. As with strength training, you'll probably see quick initial benefits from your chosen habit. But these gains are incremental over time. The longer you can dedicate yourself to the path of self-improvement, the better off you'll be.

Just like you don't want to commit to complicated behaviours in the beginning, you also don't want to take on too many new habits at once. Instead, focus your efforts on a handful of high-impact behaviours. Coming from a personal-training background, I like to see people take charge of their health and fitness through diet, exercise and recovery. But this same rule applies to other types of behaviours too: learning a musical instrument, spending less time online, reading or whatever.

Pick a few habits you want to build, then focus on adhering to them for at least two months. The habits shouldn't be so complicated that two months won't be enough to get you a long way towards having them fully ingrained. Remember that you can scale up your commitment once you've built the initial habit. It's easier to go from working out three times a week to four times a week than it is to go from zero workouts a week to four.

Think about how you can use these three ideas in your own life. Take the habit loop and see what cues could make new habits easier to build. Use the two-minute rule to commit to small behaviours – ones you can stick to when the shit hits the fan. And above all else, remember that this takes time. Don't try to become Superman overnight; build up gradually – you'll get where you're going if you keep pushing.

And speaking of habits, you don't just have to be concerned with your good ones. You also have to be vigilant against bad ones developing. If you're not careful, you can quickly become addicted to some negative behaviour that gives you short-term pleasure at the expense of long-term success. And one of the most common addictions modern men deal with? It's none other than porn.

Overcoming addiction to porn

On your journey to becoming a modern warrior, you're probably going to experience some setbacks. You'll feel dissatisfied with the process, as if things aren't happening quickly enough, and maybe you'll even become disillusioned. You might decide that there are some things you can't change about yourself or your

STRONGER MIND, STRONGER BODY, STRONGER LIFE

life, no matter how hard you try. And if you let these feelings take hold, it's easy to fall prey to something that promises to be a quick and easy fix for whatever you're missing.

If you lack confidence, you might turn to alcohol or outward displays of anger to overcompensate for this weakness. If you feel bored and purposeless, you might seek refuge in reality TV, social media, video games and other mind-numbing activities. And if you lack any kind of meaningful intimacy in your life, you might turn to porn to fill that void.

Maybe you've struggled with some or all of these at some point in your life already. They're not always problems that arise after you've begun to improve your situation – often, they're things you carry with you from a bad time in your past.

CASE STUDY: MY OWN ADDICTION

I've had difficulties of my own. Specifically, I was addicted to porn for several years. As a child, I struggled a lot with anxiety. I remember nights when my parents would head out for a meal together and leave me in the care of my grandmother. I had no reason to worry, but I'd lie awake in bed, wondering if they would be killed in a car crash on the way home. I wouldn't sleep until I heard the door open and I knew they were safe.

I had the same anxiety in other areas of my life too, particularly as I got older. I was never a big one for team sports, but looking back, I know now that I put myself under way too much pressure to perform. Too afraid of messing up and embarrassing myself in front of my friends, I wouldn't even try. And once I hit a certain age, that anxiety manifested in another important area of a man's life – romantic relationships.

Like a lot of teenage boys, I talked a big game. Around the lads, I was the man. We'd be talking about our conquests and I'd boast I'd been with a particular girl the night before. But the truth was, I hadn't. My need to impress my friends forced my back against the wall and I thought the only way out was to pretend I had much more experience than I actually had.

I'll spare you the gory details, but let's just say my first few sexual encounters were… disappointing. Once again, anxiety stopped me from relaxing and enjoying the moment. And with a few bad experiences under my belt, my anxiety had even more fuel to sustain itself. I didn't know how to articulate it back then, but I felt as if I would never be enough for a woman. As if there was no point in even trying.

This anxiety put me down a dark path for many years. The thought of facing the prison I had built for myself was terrifying. Instead, I numbed the pain by drinking too much, driving too fast and generally doing whatever I could to take my mind off my own inadequacies. To my friends, I seemed like the life of the party, but on the inside, I was dying.

Despite my best efforts to ignore them, I still had the same urges as other men. No matter that I had too much shit in my head to truly act on them. So what was the next logical step? Porn. Lots and lots of porn.

Like most young men, I had dabbled in porn for many years before I became addicted. I suppose years of anxiety and poor experiences all snowballed until it seemed like my best option.

My particular poison of choice was using chat rooms. Adult video chat rooms, just so we're clear. I had sound, visuals, access to a different partner at the click of a button – in my head, it was almost a substitute for the real thing.

What had been an occasional indulgence turned into an everyday habit. I remember staying up until 5am using these chat rooms, desperately chasing some high I could never quite achieve. Then I'd head out for work just a few hours later and wonder if people knew how broken I was on the inside.

This story has a predictable ending. When you're constantly performing on video for strangers, there's always a danger of someone taking advantage of the situation. In my case, one of my partners had recorded videos of our sessions together. And before I knew it, these videos were circulating online. It didn't take long before they were in places where my family and friends could see them.

I was horrified when I found out what was going on. Something I thought would never come to light was now exposed for all the world to see. Tremendously fucking embarrassing, to be honest. But despite how painful this was, it was also the wakeup call I had been waiting for.

For years, I had been sleepwalking through life. I kept myself numb with alcohol and porn, too afraid to open my eyes. But now I was awake.

It took time, but I managed to overcome my problems through dedicating myself to the process. Therapy was a great help (and I recommend it for anyone who needs it – no macho bullshit). Having a strong support network around me also helped. So did committing to exercising and eating healthily – fitness was an anchor for me at my worst times.

Because I've had this experience, I have a particular perspective on porn. It might be different to yours, but I'd like to share it with you; if nothing else, it will give you something to think about.

Sexual desires are part of being human. Even more so, in the context of this book, they're part of being a man. Having a high sex drive is a side effect of high testosterone levels (which can be a blessing or a curse, depending on the situation). These desires can lead people to do great things, and terrible things too.

In your efforts to attract a mate, you could work on building yourself into the best man you can be. To become more appealing to others, you might improve your fitness, become more socially fluent, learn interesting skills, get a handle on your finances etc. On the other end of the scale, if you believe that no partner could ever want you, you could be drawn to do awful things. Assault, rape, mass murder: the crimes arising from mistaken beliefs around sexuality and relationships are horrifying.

At our core, we're tribal creatures. We crave deep connection with people, meaningful relationships that add to our lives. Our mental health is largely dependent on these bonds. Without them, we feel like we're missing something. And where this gap exists, distractions rush in to numb the pain. These distractions take many forms. They may be substances such as alcohol or other drugs. They may be books, movies and stories (real or fake) that offer us an emotional high and a voyeur's perspective on what life should look like. And they can take the form of porn.

Porn is one of the most insidious drugs in existence today. It's not socially acceptable like alcohol, but it's an unspoken truth that a huge proportion of people have encountered it in their lives. In my experience, many men tend to struggle with it.

Our brains run on a cocktail of feel-good chemicals, arising whenever we achieve something of significance. Landing a big promotion at work, getting a great score in an exam, winning an athletic event, seeing a child perform in their school play – and yes, having sex with someone we have a meaningful connection with. These are all moments of significance that give us a hit of serotonin, dopamine and other mood-boosting hormones. As tribal creatures, we want to be connected to others, and porn offers us a shortcut. It's the easy way to achieve that same elated state without any hassle, heartbreak or everyday strains a relationship will bring.

When we masturbate too often, we rewire our brain to forget the true meaning behind our basic human impulses. Rather than recognising them as a signal to go out, improve ourselves and attract a partner we can be truly happy with, we rely on the instant gratification of watching sex taking place on a screen.

Twenty or thirty years ago, pornographic materials were much less prevalent than they are today. Using porn was something that took place behind closed doors, away from the eyes of judgemental friends, family and society at large. Nowadays, with the advent of the internet, the entire world of earthly desires is at our fingertips. We can see any kind of woman (or man) imaginable take off their clothes, pose and perform to our heart's content. We can choose from millions of videos, watch untold hours of footage, seek out live performers in chat rooms, pay for specially commissioned material... anything we want. In the span of an hour, we can see more naked bodies than our ancestors would have experienced in their lifetimes. And now, with modern technology, we can even strap on a virtual reality headset and pretend we're really there.

When you truly think about it, how could this possibly have any good effects on your mind? And furthermore, how could seeing someone reduced to nothing more than a hole (a vehicle for your own fulfilment) be good for you? The short answer is it couldn't.

Porn and masturbation are a poor substitute for their real-life equivalents. Rather than sharing an experience with someone you have a deep connection with, all you get is a few seconds of pleasure and the resulting dip that comes with realising you're alone. In an effort to recapture the instant high you experienced the first few times you used porn, your tastes may get wilder. You may need more and more extreme material to get off. And before long, what was once novel becomes familiar and the cycle begins all over again.

If you think that using porn to get you aroused on a regular basis won't have an impact on your sex life, you're blind to reality. And if you find it difficult to get aroused, you could end up being unable to perform when it matters. This has knock-on effects on your confidence in the bedroom. You may start to shy away from sexual encounters, preferring to express yourself in an environment where you can't be shamed or judged – in a room, by yourself.

Going from 0 to 100 takes time, as does moving in the opposite direction. You won't notice the negative effects in the short term, but in the long run? I and many other men have all seen the negative effects of excessive masturbation and porn use:

- Loss of sex drive

- Loss of drive in general

- Worsening mental health

- Lack of focus

- Less motivation to hit the gym

And the list goes on.

It's human nature to look for the easy way out. Our ancestors didn't survive by being hyperactive fools who burned off all their energy and then dropped dead; they survived thanks to the driving force of their basest biological instinct: to procreate. This urge gave them the critical edge they needed to thrive.

When you give yourself the easy way out of porn, you start to lose that edge. Your creativity, productivity, determination and zest for life all take a hit. As your brain learns to expect instant gratification, working to achieve long-term goals loses all meaning. Push far enough in this direction and you're left as little more than a lab rat, a slave to your basest urges.

You might be thinking, *That doesn't really sound like me. I don't use porn that much – that sounds like someone else's problem.* And you might be right. Maybe you manage your relationship with porn just fine. Maybe you feel it doesn't have an impact on the way you interact with people, your love life, your career or your fitness. The vast majority of men don't have any visible problems with porn. Most use it occasionally, log off, and then don't think about it again.

However, it's easy to let problems creep up on you. And when porn offers so little genuine value to your life while potentially holding you back so much, why not err on the side of caution? Here's an easy way for you to test yourself…

Go porn-free for ninety days

If you're currently in a relationship, this shouldn't be too hard. If you're single, it may be more challenging, but still doable – if you don't have a problem. But if you do have any issues with porn, they will soon reveal themselves. You'll catch yourself pulling up a site without thinking when you're alone and you'll wonder how deep that habit goes. You may struggle to resist the urge as the days pass, but over time, the urge *will* diminish. The neural pathways you've built around porn use will become disused and their pull will weaken.

A well-developed man has a healthy relationship with his sexuality. If you allow your appetite to define you – to guide your behaviours – and you make bad decisions based on it, you'll suffer. Most people won't have the same trouble I had with porn, but my perspective has given me an insight into how damaging it can be. I don't demonise it (or people who use it), but I view it like other addictions. How much value will it contribute to your life? To your legacy? To your vision of becoming a better man?

These are questions you need to ask yourself. And if you come to the conclusion that you need help, don't be afraid to reach out. Counselling can help you overcome addiction to porn, as can having a strong support network of friends, family and like-minded individuals.

I firmly believe that a man should be self-reliant. If you're a slave to porn and the instant pleasure it promises, you'll stunt your growth as a person. If you can take the energy you previously squandered on porn and apply it to self-improvement, you'll soon find that your career, your social life and your fitness will improve. And when all these pieces fall into place, you'll have an easier time than before attracting a great partner into your life.

The life you want and the deep relationships you need can be yours. But if you stay mired in dysfunction, they'll forever elude you. Take the time now to get a grasp on your sexuality before it causes real problems for you. And remember, porn addiction is just like any other addiction. Maybe your problem is alcohol, gambling, the internet, social media or hard drugs like cocaine. Whatever the case may be, know this:

You can change. It all starts with taking that first step.

We've covered a lot of ground in the first section of this book, and with good reason – getting control over your mind is the first thing you must do to become a modern warrior. Your mind will determine whether your journey is one of success or abject failure. Without taking the time to build mastery in this area, you'll eternally struggle to achieve even a fraction of what you're capable of.

Some of the mental shifts we've covered in this section are subtle, but powerful. Perhaps they're not too different to how you view the world already. Some of them may even seem like common sense. But there is a difference between knowing and understanding. Most people know everything they need to know about how to do something, eg lose weight, improve their fitness, land a new job. But despite this knowledge, they still can't succeed, because they don't understand how their mind works. They haven't taken the time to internalise the key perspectives that would help them see the world in a new light. They haven't learned how to harness their willpower, build better habits and hack their motivation. They don't understand that their ability to reframe everything life throws at them could mean the difference between success and failure.

To do things is not complicated, but it certainly is difficult. You'll have to put in real effort to master your mind. There will be times when you question why you're even bothering with cold showers, meditation sessions or pushing yourself one step further. But learning to engage in the process of doing all these things is how you will succeed in the long run.

The path of the strong welcomes all travellers, but it's not an easy route for those who lack the conviction to keep walking, even when night gathers and you can't see through the darkness before you. In these times, your mind will be your greatest asset; the light that leads the way through the night, bringing you closer and closer to your destination. Spend the time now and learn how to master your mind. Take what we've covered here, run with it, then add your own learnings into the mix. Becoming a stronger you isn't an easy process, but the results are worth it. And getting your mind right is 80% of the battle.

Now that we've covered the concept of a strong mind in detail, it's time to turn our attention to the next piece of the puzzle: the strong body.

PART TWO
THE STRONG BODY

'It is a shame for a man to grow old
without seeing the beauty and strength
of which his body is capable.'
— Socrates

6
Strength First

Welcome to the training section of this book! Here, you'll find the essential techniques you'll need to create real changes in your health and fitness. While I haven't covered every possible topic in detail, I've provided you with the most critical material – the stuff that will have the biggest impact on your life.

Your powerful mind is the driver. Your body is the vehicle. Both need the other to realise their full potential. A Formula 1 driver on a pedal bike will lose out to a casual driver in a Bugatti Veyron every time. But take that professional and put him in a car built for speed? He'll dominate the competition. It's the same way with your mind and body. Getting your mind right is the first, most important step. Once you've taken care of this, you can focus on the second part of the process – building your body into a weapon that will serve you well in all you do.

Your health is your wealth. The most driven and dedicated person will struggle to hit peak performance if they're constantly sick, aching or tired. At the same time, you don't have to build your entire life around maintaining a supermodel's 5% body fat percentage.

Coming from a personal-training background, I've helped many people achieve a broad spectrum of goals. Weight loss, muscle gain, enhanced athletic performance, better appearance – you name it, someone has looked for help with it. Most people don't care about setting a world record in their sport, competing as a professional bodybuilder or walking around like a contest-ready fitness model. If those are your goals, more power to you. But just be warned that they'll require a lot of energy to achieve. And given that you only have a certain amount of time in the day, you might reasonably say that you don't want to pursue these goals. That's perfectly fine. I always encourage people to go after what they care about, not what they think they should care about.

Just so we're all on the same page:

- You don't need to train for two hours a day, six days a week to build a powerful, attractive physique
- You don't need to rigidly adhere to three meals a day of chicken, rice and broccoli to lose weight
- You don't have to forego getting enough sleep to have any chance at achieving your goals

These are all extreme examples, but they reinforce my underlying point:

You can achieve great results with a reasonable approach.

By that, I mean that you can easily be in the top 5–10% in whatever area you care about by following an intelligent plan, adopting some key habits and committing yourself to the process. Whether you want to get bigger, smaller, stronger, build endurance or just get fit for a recreational sport, you can do it. And it doesn't have to be painful or complicated.

The strong man knows that building a healthy, strong body will serve him well on the path. But with everything his mission demands of him, he has to be intelligent in his approach. He can't hope to overcome a lack of knowledge or dedication by giving all his energy away freely; instead, he has to be strategic about the process.

In this section of the book, we'll cover everything you need to know to build a great level of strength, fitness and health, so you can ensure your mind isn't trapped in your body like a Formula 1 driver on a push bike. Specifically, we're going to talk about:

- Why building strength is one of the best things to focus on as a man and how to go about it, including the most fundamental truth of all exercise programming (pay attention to this, and pretty much any workout program will get you good results)

- The tools of transformation you'll encounter on your journey

- The main exercises you need to be familiar with to build world-class fitness

- The most important programming principles you need to understand to achieve great results (frequency, volume, intensity and rest periods)

- The basics of high-performance nutrition – how to eat for maximum energy and peak performance

- The key supplements you can take to make your journey easier and my views on steroids

- Recovery – why sleep matters, how to optimise it and how to recover in general

The information in this section is distilled from my years as a personal trainer, coaching hundreds of people to achieve their goals. What you'll see here are the gems I've accumulated over these years – putting them into practice is sure to shortcut your journey towards gaining mastery over your body. If you're ready to develop your body into the weapon you need it to be, then read on.

Training

I'd like to talk now about the one quality you need to focus on above all else. This quality is strength – a common term, but one that's often inaccurately defined.

For our purposes, strength is defined as 'the ability of a muscle or muscle group to exert maximum force against resistance'. We can easily envision strength as the maximum weight we can lift on an exercise. For instance, someone who can bench press 50 kg for one repetition is weaker than someone who can bench press 100 kg for one repetition. But strength is not limited solely to the weight room. Depending on the career you're in, you may need strength throughout your day (particularly if you work in construction or some other manual job). Having the physical strength to get yourself out of bed in the morning is what separates you from a bed-bound patient in a nursing home. Strength propels you up that steep flight of stairs when you're carrying six bags of shopping and rooting for your keys.

Being strong is correlated with being muscular too. While the relationship between the two is not perfectly linear, it's generally safe to say that a bigger person (all else being equal) will be stronger than a smaller one.

Strength matters because it lays the foundation for everything else. Being stronger makes your life easier, helps you to look better and gives you an innate sense of confidence. Knowing that you're able to handle heavier weights than you could a month, three months or a year ago is tangible proof of your progress – something many of us miss in other areas of life.

When I'm creating training programs for clients, I like to make sure I've covered my bases by addressing the four pillars of physical fitness:

- Strength
- Endurance
- Mobility
- Motor control

While all four of these qualities are covered in all of my programs, strength is usually the priority. This is because strength training has the greatest impact on everything else. And assuming you don't focus on strength to the exclusion of all else, you'll notice there's plenty of carryover to everything you do in the gym.

How to build strength

Broadly speaking, there are two factors that contribute to how strong you are:

1. How much muscle you have

2. How efficient your nervous system is at using this muscle

To understand what these two factors are, let's imagine a car. In this example, how much muscle you have = the size of the fuel tank, and the efficiency of your nervous system = your car's fuel consumption. A car that has a 100-litre fuel tank has the potential to go further than a car with a 50-litre tank, but won't go as far as a car with a 150-litre tank. Likewise, a car that does 30 miles per gallon won't get as far as a car that does 60 miles per gallon. So a car with a 50-litre tank that does 60 miles per gallon would theoretically go just as far as the 100-litre car doing 30 miles per gallon.

If we want to improve the performance of the car, we have two options: increase the capacity of the fuel tank or increase its efficiency. If we increase the efficiency of our 100-litre car from 30 miles per gallon to 60 miles per gallon, then we can travel twice as far on the same amount of fuel. Likewise, if we increase the capacity of the tank from 100 litres to 200 litres, we'll go twice as far without having to worry about efficiency increases at all. Simple enough, yeah?

Your body is the same. If you want to get stronger, you need to either get bigger (ie increase your muscle mass) or get better at using what you've already got. Of course, you don't have to pick one or the other – this is just to illustrate our point.

So strength has both a physical component and a skill-based component. The physical side is how much muscle you have, while the skill-based component is how efficient you are at a particular movement. Returning to our earlier example of bench pressing, the person benching 50 kg has two paths they can take to increase their lift:

1. They can get stronger overall and focus on increasing their muscle mass

2. They can focus on getting better at benching, doing the lift frequently, making technique adjustments etc

When people first start lifting, they frequently report big initial strength gains (referred to as 'newbie gains'). Novices can often add weight to the bar every single session for extended periods. But we now know that there are two ways they could be building strength – either they're building muscle, or they're getting better at using what they already have.

Muscle-building is a slow physiological process. For most people, a 7–9 kg muscle gain in their first year of lifting would be brilliant progress (obvious exceptions apply, but this is for the most part). In reality, the rapid gains they see at the start of a new program are down to the fact that their body is getting better at whatever they're doing.

Generally, it's quicker to get better at something specific than it is to build the muscle required to be stronger overall. But if you're interested in getting stronger, then you don't need to specialise in a handful of exercises. You just need to work through a variety of movements as part of an intelligently designed system.

One of the biggest training mistakes I see people make is thinking that they have to max out all the time to build strength. Honestly, nothing could be further from the truth. While hitting a max lift and moving a huge weight is good for your ego (and for your social media likes, if you're so inclined), it's only a display of strength – a demonstration of what you've already built. Constant maxing out doesn't help most people to build strength. Unless you happen to be genetically suited to this style of training (wide frame, thick joints that can handle the stress), you're better off building your strength in a variety of rep ranges.

We'll talk about sets and reps in a later chapter – for now, just remember that you don't need to max out all the time to build strength.

The most fundamental training principle

If I could only teach you one training principle, it would be this: your body adapts to the stresses you put on it. And when you understand what this means, you'll know that the implications of this fundamental biological truth go far beyond the realm of training. They underpin your entire life.

Whatever kind of body you have right now is the body that your lifestyle (up until this point) has required. If you've spent the last ten years sitting on the couch doing nothing more taxing than watching Netflix or scrolling through your Instagram feed, your body will reflect that. In contrast, if you have spent the past ten years training hard multiple times per week, your body will be proof of that too.

Think of what happens when you break an arm or a leg. The cast goes on for six to eight weeks, and when it comes off, the muscle in that limb has wasted away from lack of use. It's only through starting to use it again (and making a conscious effort to build yourself back up) that you restore function.

The process of muscles wasting away is known as atrophy. The process they undergo to grow bigger is known as hypertrophy. But building bigger muscles is a biologically expensive process. Unless your lifestyle demands that you possess a certain level of strength and fitness, your body has little reason to maintain it.

The reason why it's hard to stay fit or muscular without working hard for it is because we (as humans) are wired to run efficiently. Back in our hunter-gatherer days, food was scarce – we never knew where the next meal was coming from. Having to lug around a ton of extra muscle mass was wasteful. All we could afford to carry was the amount required to get our next meal – anything else was impractical.

While we don't have to hunt for our dinner anymore, our genetics remain largely unchanged from those days. So if your level of strength and fitness is lower than you'd like it to be, look at your lifestyle. You'll probably find that the demands you've imposed on your body in the recent past are a mirror image of where you currently are physically.

Your lifestyle sends signals to your body about what it needs to be able to do to survive. So what does effective signalling look like? We'll dive into this more in later chapters, but for now, think of it like this. You need to send signals to your body that tell it you want more muscle and less fat. If you subject your body to hard, intelligent strength training (ie tell it that it needs to be able to exert a great amount of force on a repeated basis), you'll send a good signal. If you eat a well-balanced diet that promotes leanness and muscularity (not one that encourages your body to store extra calories in preparation for a hard winter), you'll send a good signal. If you go out and run for countless miles, week after week, you'll send a signal to your body that you need to be efficient for this. And as you can imagine, people who run fast marathons don't tend to be very muscular.

Simply put – your diet and exercise routine have to send the right signal to your body. Without putting an appropriate stress on your system, you'll never get better. But that's the crucial point there: it has to be an *appropriate* level of stress.

I touch on this again in later chapters, but I've never found maxing out day after day, week after week in the gym to be a good approach for most natural lifters. Unless you happen to put on muscle easily or you have a frame that can take that sort of punishment (wide build, thick joints etc), then it's not a smart path to follow. On the other end of the spectrum, performing the most gruelling dumbbell circuit in the world with 2 kg dumbbells will only be effective so long as 2 kg is a challenging weight for you (and for most people, this won't be long). You need to find the sweet spot between too much and too little stress. When I'm writing programs for my clients, I like to see them performing a particular exercise 3–10 times (repetitions) per 'set' for most of their heavier movements, with higher repetition ranges (10–20) being used for their accessory work and extras. (There will be more on sets, reps and the equipment to use in later chapters.)

Smart programming is all about knowing when to go for heavy weights and when to back off and do more reps, and the devil is often in the details. This is a tricky subject, but honestly – if you get a grasp of the fundamentals, you'll be miles ahead of the people floundering around, stuck using the same weights for weeks and months on end. And this principle – that you adapt to whatever appropriate stress you put yourself under – extends far beyond the gym.

We're all familiar with the concept of a comfort zone. If you've ever had to get better at anything in your life, there was probably a time where you had to do something that wasn't comfortable for you. Our comfort zones protect us when we need it, but they can also hold us back from success. That's why it's important to both embrace and challenge your comfort zone when trying to achieve a goal. Even for someone who's never really exercised before, the idea of going for a 30–40 minute walk wouldn't sound too bad; but going to a weightlifting gym? Way too intimidating.

Although both are forms of exercise, there's a key difference between them: one is inside their comfort zone, and the other, outside. It's important when establishing goals to remember that it's in the sweet spot – the middle between those two extremes of comfort – where the magic happens.

Constantly exposing yourself to appropriate amounts of stress will build a body you can be proud of. Applying this lesson outside the gym will allow you to live a life you love. The alternative is to stay in your comfort zone, choose to live an easy life, and let your fitness levels decline in response to the demands you place on yourself. This is more comfortable in the short term, but it leads you to ruin in the long term.

Don't be afraid of stress. It will make you into the strong man you want to be.

7
The Tools of Transformation

When you first set out on your health and fitness journey, it's easy to get confused. There are as many diet and training protocols floating around as you can count. You're likely to see the talking heads on morning TV shows lifting water bottles, stretching rubber bands and showing off their flash running shoes. Huge men lifting colossal weights in documentaries about steroid use. Runners huffing and puffing their way to victory in a gruelling long-distance event. With all these options laid out in front of you, how the fuck do you find what works? How do you know what tools to use?

The truth is, pretty much anything will work if you do it hard enough. That said, we're focusing on building strength here, not being able to run marathons, complete loads of random circuits or lift a heavy weight once (and then lie down after). Your goal as a strong man is to build the kind of strength that makes your life better – that helps you look better, feel better and perform better. And to achieve that, certain tools are better than others.

Depending on your athletic background, you may not be familiar with the inside of a gym. Walking into one for the first time can be an intimidating experience for anyone. Gyms can be crowded, noisy, confusing and downright off-putting. And even if you find a great place that's welcoming, there's no guarantee that you'll actually know how to use the equipment in front of you.

My aim with this chapter is to give you a broad overview of the kinds of tools you can use to change your body and take charge of your health and fitness. This is not an exhaustive list; rather, it's my take on the most popular options you'll have in front of you.

Let's start with the elephant in the room – free weights.

Free weights

Free weights are a common fixture of pretty much any decent gym. If you're in a chain gym, odds are that they'll take up a lot less space than the machines or cardio equipment (we'll discuss both of these later on in this chapter), but they'll be there.

When I talk about free weights, I'm primarily referring to:

• Dumbbells

• Barbells and weight plates

• Benches

• Power/squat racks

I'd also include stuff like dip stations and pull-up bars in the mix as they're both valuable pieces of kit that are massively helpful in building real-world strength.

We call these 'free weights' because we control them independently, without any external stabilisation. This is what distinguishes them from exercise machines, the sort you might see around any gym floor. (If you're unfamiliar with them, don't worry! They'll be covered in greater detail later.)

For example, consider the difference between a barbell bench press and a chest press machine. With the bench press, you're forced to control the bar throughout the movement, which means that you employ more muscle fibres. With the chest press, the movement is stabilised for you. This means that you can often use more weight (although not always) at the expense of being forced to move in a fixed range of motion.

Dumbbells add an additional element of stabilisation to many movements. Consider a dumbbell bench press vs a barbell bench press. When you're doing the dumbbell movement, you have to control each hand independently, instead of having them both in a fixed position relative to one another (as is the case when you use a barbell).

Free weights are great because they're versatile. With a single barbell, a couple of adjustable dumbbell handles and enough weight plates, you can create a workout that effectively trains your entire body. In contrast, you'd need dozens of machines to achieve the same result (ultimate home gym contraptions are a waste of money). This makes free weights an ideal choice for someone looking to set up a garage gym, provided you account for safety.

Free weights are also great because they help you to train the most important quality you need to focus on as a strong man: strength. Barbells and dumbbells are both easy to load precisely, so you know exactly how much you're lifting in any given exercise. With this in mind, it's simple to measure your progress over time, allowing you to determine whether you're getting stronger, staying the same or declining.

A common misconception is that free weights are more dangerous than machines. While it's true that people get injured while weight training, this is nearly always down to poor technique and not being able to read the warning signs of an impending injury. If you know how to perform the movements correctly and exercise common sense, you'll be fine.

Free weights are at the core of my programming because they're simply the most effective tool for most guys to achieve the results they desire. Unless you have specific athletic goals that warrant the use of other protocols (eg you're a runner, you play a sport or you're training for an event), spend the majority of your workout with free weights.

Machines

Instead of using a traditional bench-and-barbell or dumbbells, some gym-goers opt to use exercise machines for their workout. Although these machines may seem daunting at first, they're mechanically very simple. Most exercise machines are built for completion of only a single exercise, and can be used after just a few minutes of research or instruction.

For that reason (their ease of access and use) machines can be very useful. Although not as versatile as free weights, they can be a godsend for some. For instance, if you're recovering from an injury or wanting to rehab one muscle group in particular, machines can allow you to train that area in isolation to everything else (we'll talk more about isolation exercises in a later chapter).

Machines typically take up a lot of floor space in gyms. Because each piece of equipment is used for only one exercise, gyms need a large variety of them.

One of the key features of machines is that they remove the need for you to stabilise the weight throughout the movement. By limiting you to a fixed range of motion, they enable you to move heavier weights than you could with the equivalent free-weight exercise. This can be good or bad, depending on the situation: more weight = more muscle fibre recruitment, but lack of stabilisation = lack of real-world relevance.

I incorporate machine exercises into my programming on a case-by-case basis, depending on what my clients need. For instance, a leg curl machine can be useful for training your hamstrings directly – a muscle group that's often neglected in standard training programs. I also like to work in leg presses and leg extensions, simply because they're good exercises for isolating the legs.

Overall, machines are a valuable tool when incorporated as part of a well-structured plan.

Cardio equipment

Cardio equipment will dominate a large amount of floor space in pretty much any standard gym. To be clear, when we talk about cardio equipment, we're talking about:

- Treadmills

- Exercise bikes

- Cross trainers

- Stair steppers

- Rowing machines

- Ski ergs

And everything else designed to get your heart rate up and your sweat flowing. You could even throw in stuff like skipping ropes here (although their application tends to be a bit different).

Cardio equipment is a popular choice for anyone looking to lose weight or get 'fitter'. When people think of someone who's 'fit', they usually think of someone who can run for miles on end, pedal for days or do anything physical for a long time without getting tired. Your personal definition of fitness may be a bit different, but that's the general perception people have.

Using cardio equipment is straightforward. Apart from the initial confusion any first-timer might experience, it's fairly intuitive. Cardio equipment allows you to tailor your workout to your current fitness levels. For example, decent treadmills offer a variety of speed and incline options; exercise bikes and cross trainers have adjustable resistance. This allows you to gauge your progress over time, ensuring you're getting better over the weeks and months you spend using them.

But do these pieces of equipment help you to grow stronger? The answer depends on your goals. For the purpose of general strength development, you don't need to put in hours of running, cycling or otherwise moving. For that goal, spending your time with targeted strength-training exercises is the best approach.

Cardio equipment does exactly what it says on the tin. It targets your cardiovascular system (your heart and lungs) directly, which has numerous health benefits. While this probably isn't a huge concern to you if you're a young guy, the fact is that four of the top five causes of death relate to the function of your heart and lungs, so it's certainly worth paying attention to as you age. And if you're trying to lose weight, intelligently incorporating cardio into your routine is a good move.

When creating programs for my personal-training clients, I tend to use cardio equipment for warm-ups and extra work for those who need it. While I believe that training your cardiovascular system is important, I don't necessarily think that you have to use a treadmill to do so. In fact, proper weight training with shortened rest intervals (which we'll discuss in further detail later on in this book) can be effective in helping you to build strength and fitness at the same time.

Everything else

Now let's talk about everything else you might encounter in a gym, see on Instagram or otherwise come across on your fitness journey. This includes:

- Sandbags

- Kettlebells

- Kegs

- Tyres

- Sledgehammers

- Battle ropes

- TRX systems

- Prowlers

- Sledges

The appeal of these items is obvious. People love novelty and variety. They're attracted to strange-looking tools, eager to find out how they can incorporate them into their routine in an effective manner. But the truth is these tools are just tools. They're effective for achieving certain outcomes, but ineffective for others.

Take sandbags, for instance. In case you're unfamiliar, a sandbag is exactly what it sounds like: a bag filled with sand, gravel, salt or some other substance. When you lift the sandbag, the contents shift around, making the movement much more challenging (as it requires additional stabilisation, taxes your grip etc). Using equipment like this is great for seeing how you stack up against something that's not as balanced and easily assessed as a barbell. It can also be a useful tool to incorporate into conditioning workouts. While it's not the best choice for building gym strength, it can be great for building functional strength. This is because it takes emphasis away from your bigger, stronger muscle groups and places it on the smaller ones needed to stabilise the movement.

In the real world, these muscles are very important, whether you're helping a friend move house, performing on the sports pitch or doing anything apart from lifting a barbell. Although someone who uses sandbags as their primary strength-building tool may lag behind a free-weight user in terms of maximum strength on certain movements, they could function just as well when it comes to the crunch.

The same goes for everything else I listed too. I often incorporate TRX exercises into my programming. Kettlebells are great for certain movements. Pretty much everything is effective when it's used properly, but that's the key point: it has to be used properly.

Don't get distracted by novel pieces of equipment. Focus on hammering the basics hard, track your progress and stay dedicated. You won't regret it.

8
The Movements

You've made it to this point in Part Two – you're doing well! We've covered a lot of ground so far; we've discussed the importance of strength, why it should matter to you and the various tools you can use to build it. But what we haven't done yet is look at the movements to use to train strength in detail. If you're a seasoned gym-goer, you're probably familiar with a lot of the exercises we'll discuss in this chapter, but if you're new to fitness, or you're looking to level up your knowledge and ensure you're covering all your bases, then read on.

A tool is only as useful as you can make it. A guitar can produce show-stopping music or an ear-splitting din, depending on who's playing it. A car can be a mode of transport or a deadly weapon. And a barbell can be a powerful tool of self-transformation or an accident waiting to happen. Each of the tools of transformation we discussed in the previous chapter are practically worthless unless you know how to use them properly. And how do you use them properly? You use them to train specific movement patterns that hit your major muscle groups effectively.

There's a lot of overlap in what people think is important. While the nitty-gritty details may differ, the fact is that certain movements form the cornerstone of any effective training program. We can argue all day whether this exercise is better than that one, or if one variation is superior to another, but in the end, as long as we're training the movement pattern in a safe, loadable, easily measured way, then it's good enough.

One important thing to note here is the difference between compound movements and isolation movements. In simple terms, a compound movement involves more than one joint and works more than one muscle group. An isolation movement involves only one joint and typically works a single muscle group.

To give you a concrete example, let's consider the difference between a pull-up and a bicep curl. Pull-ups involve movement around the shoulder and elbow joints. They hit all the muscles in your upper back, your biceps, forearms and shoulders. Bicep curls, on the other hand, primarily target your biceps (it's in the name, after all).

If your aim is to build real-world strength, spend the majority of your time working compound movements. You'll make better use of your time in the gym, train your body to work together as one unit and see strength increases you couldn't see from isolation exercises alone.

That said, isolation exercises are still an important part of a well-structured routine. They allow you to focus on specific muscle groups, helping you to keep getting bigger and stronger as you progress. They're also great when it comes to isolating the muscles that you want to be bigger (relative to the rest of your frame). Think your shoulders, arms etc.

Now that's out of the way, let's talk about the movements I consider to be most important in training.

Push

No getting away from this one, lads: your push strength matters. From doing push-ups on the floor to struggling with light weight on the bench press the day you start, pushing needs to be a key focus of your program. It's pretty important.

Push movements target your chest, arms and shoulders. All of these muscles are instrumental in helping you build real strength, look better and improve your performance.

My favourite pushing exercises include push-ups, dips, overhead presses, bench presses (all variations) and tricep extensions. I include a good amount of these exercises in all the programs I write simply because they're effective, people like doing them and they're pretty easy to get the hang of.

Now that we've talked all about pushing exercises, let's move on to...

Pull

It's important to mention that most people focus too much on pushing exercises to the detriment of their pulling exercises (your pushing muscles are easily visible in a mirror – they're the ones you see when you're flexing for that selfie). This is a mistake. With the lives that most of us lead (working on computers, heads down, shoulders rounded forward as we tap away on our phones or keyboards), the last thing we need is to add more dysfunction on top of what's already there. To combat serious postural issues, I include a good amount of pulling exercises in every program I design.

If pushing exercises train the front half of your upper body, pulling exercises do the opposite, hitting the muscles of the back. Pulling exercises you might be familiar with are pull-ups, chin-ups, lat pulldowns, rows (of all kinds) and bicep curls.

Problematic posture is easily fixable if you put in the time with pulling movements. Assuming you employ good form throughout the movement and don't go crazy with the amount of weight you're using, you'll be able to reverse the posture-destroying effects of the modern lifestyle and set yourself up for even greater success in the long term. This doesn't just matter from a functional/health standpoint, it's also important if you're interested in looking better. Training with heavy pulling exercises helps you to build that elusive v-taper.

Now that we've covered the upper body, let's move on to the lower body.

Squat

If you've spent any time in a gym at all, you're probably familiar with squatting. Unfortunately, there's a good chance you:

- Don't do it properly

- Don't do it regularly

- Don't do it all because you think it's too dangerous

If any of those resonate with you, we need to get that straightened out right away.

When I talk about squatting, I mean exercises like front squats (squatting with the bar held in front of you), back squats (squatting with the bar held across your shoulders), pistols (squatting while standing on one leg), air squats (squatting with no additional weight) or anything like that. It's fairly self-explanatory: if it looks like you're sitting down and then standing up again, it's a squat.

A properly performed squat is no more dangerous than any other exercise you'll do. If you do them right and employ good technique, you'll be fine – assuming you exercise a little common sense. Pushing through some light cramping is fine. Pushing through an impending hernia is not.

Squatting is a crucial part of any well-formed strength routine because it works many vital areas of the body. First and foremost, it trains your legs (primarily your quads, but it also hits your hamstrings, calves and glutes). Your whole core is heavily involved because it's required to stabilise you throughout the movement. Depending on the variation you're doing, you can work even more muscles (eg your upper back is taxed by back squats).

Squats are hailed as one of the most crucial exercises you need to do if you're serious about making gains.

While I don't believe that they're magical (like a lot of lifters in days past did), I do think they're important. Squatting is practical. It gives you the kind of real-world leg strength that you can use to run faster for longer or stabilise yourself when you're pushing a heavy weight overhead. And there's nothing quite like a set of heavy squats for training your mental toughness. I incorporate squats into all my programming, and they're usually present in some form on every training day (even if it's only as a warm-up).

Squats are one of two major movement patterns that hit your lower body. Let's look at the other now.

Deadlift

If squats are the king of lower body exercises, deadlifts are ... the second king. Look, they're important – just go with me on this.

When I talk about deadlifts, I'm referring to the broad group of exercises including trap bar deadlifts (deadlifts with a special hexagonal bar), Romanian deadlifts (hamstring-heavy variant), rack pulls (deadlifts which start from a higher pulling point than the floor), and block pulls (same again). Any movement where you're raising the bar from the ground (or wherever it's resting) using the power of your hips and glutes falls into this category.

Deadlifts are an important movement because they offer real-world benefits. They strengthen your capacity to move heavy loads, increase your athletic ability (improving your sprint speed and jumping power, for instance) and help add muscle to your frame in key areas. But deadlifting, much like squatting, is an activity that many people fear because it seems risky – as if there's a high chance of injury associated with it. The fact is that deadlifting is perfectly safe when you do it correctly (assuming you have no genuine pre-existing issues).

It's also important to note that you don't have to do conventional deadlifts straight from the floor. You can substitute in trap bar deadlifts, rack pulls from mid-shin height or some other suitable alternative.

If you give deadlifts an appropriate amount of attention, you'll soon find that you can move more weight than you can on any other exercise. There's nothing quite like piling on the plates for a heavy triple and nailing it with ease. But because you can train them to heavier weights than any other exercise, deadlifts can be quite taxing to recover from. Most people don't do well deadlifting heavy weights more than once/twice a week.

Deadlifting is a crucial part of any well-written strength program. If you're interested in building a foundation of strength that will serve you in all you do, then don't neglect to work these.

Now we've covered the upper body and lower body in some detail, it's time to turn our attention to the final piece of the puzzle...

Core

Depending on how old you are or how long you've been around the fitness space, you may or may not remember the time when core training was the Holy Grail of fitness. All manner of bullshit was spewed and accepted as fact as people wobbled on balance boards, did crazy-looking movements and struggled through set after set of core exercises in an effort to get the gains they so desperately wanted.

The core training fad has died down since its heyday from 2009 to 2013, but it's still a hot topic for many people. And it's no wonder why. As a society, we've been conditioned to believe that having a six-pack is the only fitness goal that matters to a man. In our quest for that perfect set of abs, some of us fall prey to quick-fix pills, useless pieces of equipment and silly diet hacks in an effort to shortcut the process.

The truth is, getting a great set of abs is much simpler than you've been led to believe. If you want to have visible abs, it's not training you need to worry about – it's your diet. Being able to see your six-pack comes down to having a sufficiently low body fat percentage so that the abdominal muscles show through your skin.

There's a reason trainers often joke that 'abs are made in the kitchen' – it's because they really are!

But of course, the focus of this book is not solely on how you look. The strong man cares about building real, usable strength, and then enjoying the aesthetic benefit as a nice side effect.

The muscles of your core (including your abs, obliques, spinal erectors) play an important role in your strength development. Without solid core strength to fall back on, you'll be hampering your own progress and leaving the door to potential injury wide open.

The role of your core is to stabilise and support you throughout whatever movement you're doing. Whether you're squatting, deadlifting, pushing or pulling, your core is integral to doing that exercise in a safe manner. In this sense, your core acts as a bridge between your upper and lower body, allowing you to keep both in harmony as you work out.

With this key function of your core in mind, let's consider the kind of exercises that will be most effective. Don't waste time doing endless reps of sit ups, chasing the burn or following random fads that promise the world, but deliver nothing. Instead, focus on really nailing a couple of basic exercises and using those to help you achieve your goals.

The kinds of core exercises I typically put in my programs include all types of planks (an exercise where you hold something like a push-up position for as long as possible), or hanging leg raises (where you hang from a bar and lift your legs/knees at a 90-degree angle). The core also gets plenty of indirect work when you do your other movements – having to stabilise a heavy load as you're squatting or deadlifting is challenging enough to cause your body to adapt. Core work is something to do (either directly or indirectly) pretty much every day in a well-formed strength routine.

Now that we've covered the five main movements I like to prescribe, it's time to talk about...

Everything else

I know this is the second time I've used 'everything else' as a catch-all at the end of a chapter, but believe me, there's good reason why I've done this. If all you do every time you go into the gym is hit push, pull, squat, deadlift and core exercise for decent reps and sets (enough to create a stimulus, not enough to cripple you), work hard, track your progress and repeat all this two to five times a week, you'll do just fine. You'll make great gains – assuming your diet and recovery is on point.

But that kind of routine isn't perfect. There are a lot of body parts, muscles and movements not addressed in those five categories. Take your neck, for instance. If you're a collision athlete of any kind (eg you play rugby) or a competitor in a combat sport like boxing or mixed martial arts, having a strong neck is important. Or you might be a sprinter who needs extra glute and hamstring work to keep you fit for race season. You might just want to improve how you look by training specific muscle groups more than others.

Whatever the case may be, there's always the scope for adding more exercises than we've discussed so far. When writing programs, I tend to add these extras on a case-by-case basis. Different goals require different approaches. But I don't believe you can go wrong by dedicating the majority of your time and energy to building strength with the basics of pushing, pulling, squatting, deadlifting and core movements.

9
Exercise Programming

Exercise programming – in simple terms – is how your routine is put together. The exercises you do, how often you train, how you progress, your rest periods, exercise tempo, special techniques – all of these topics and more fall beneath the umbrella of programming.

Obviously, with such a wide array of factors to consider, programming can get complicated. That's why so many people are confused about how to train. The limitless number of options out there mean that they often don't move past the paralysis by analysis stage in their journey.

In my experience, the average guy who wants to look good, be strong for real life and healthy enough to do whatever he wants to doesn't need much complexity in his training. And that's why many non-competitive trainees simply do whatever they've seen other people do, or what they heard from a friend, family member or internet fitness personality. And often, this works just fine.

Depending on the source you're getting your information from, you could get lucky. Maybe the person you're following knows a lot about fitness and proper programming. But it may be a good idea to ensure they have some actual qualifications as well as real results – not just one or the other.

You can also get unlucky. I believe that's why gyms everywhere are filled with people who struggle to get the results they want. They learned enough from their chosen source of information to get started, but not enough to reach their goals. When they eventually run into an unforeseen obstacle, they don't have the tools they require to overcome it. Then they plateau, remaining at the same level for months and years at a time. Often they get disillusioned and quit altogether – not surprising when they never get the results they're looking for.

If you're lucky enough to be blessed with good genetics, then pretty much any workout will work well for you. You won't need to pay attention to what experts recommend – you can go in and just lift, letting the results come naturally. Chances are that if you fall into this category, you'll already know about it.

Here's my quick take on programming. Training in accordance with a few fundamental principles will allow you to get 90% of the results you could possibly get from any program. As long as you abide by the basic tenets of effective exercise programming, there's no need to sweat the small stuff. We can debate all day whether you should rest for sixty seconds or ninety seconds, but ultimately, it doesn't really matter.

When you see a new program put out by your favourite coach, you're seeing something they've designed with an end goal in mind. It represents just one potential path to that goal. It is not the only way to do it – far from it. There are a million different programs out there with a million success stories, a million failures and a million modifications to boot. You can get stronger using barbells, dumbbells, kettlebells, machines, your bodyweight or simply performing manual labour. You can get more aerobically fit by running, swimming, walking, cycling, and even by finding a willing partner to spend some quality time with (note: this one comes highly recommended).

With so many different methods to choose from, it's easy to see why people feel intimidated. But there's no reason to be. The variety of choices before you can inspire you, not scare you. It shows that you can achieve your goals using any number of methods. But the keys to progress remain the same, no matter how you choose to obtain them.

Within certain parameters, everything works. The criteria by which you determine something has worked (ie does it achieve its main goal?) may change, but the most important piece of the puzzle is – and always will be – your commitment to the process.

The fundamentals are your foundation – the optimisation is merely icing on the cake, so to speak. In the long term, working out in accordance with the principles I'm going to outline in this chapter will get you all the results you need. I'll touch on each of the most important aspects of proper programming, giving you all the information you require to understand the why behind various programs. Each section starts with my top principle(s) to reap the benefits of this knowledge.

Training frequency

Principle: training frequently is better for both strength and muscle gain, but if it's not realistic for you to be in the gym six days a week, do what you can. I personally like to see trainees in the gym three to five days a week as that's a nice balance between reaping the benefits of high-frequency training and fitting in with the rest of their lives.

There are many high-frequency training methods out there. One of the most famous is known as the Bulgarian Method, so called because it was the system used by Bulgarian weightlifters in the seventies and eighties to dominate the global strength scene.[1] Other popular high-frequency methods include Pavel Tsatsouline's Grease the Groove approach to strength-building[2] and Dan John's Easy Strength.[3] Both of these programs are based on the notion that strength is a skill and the best way to build this skill is by practising frequently.

At the same time, there are some common low-frequency methods out there too. Dorian Yates (six-time Mr Olympia winner) popularised infrequent high-intensity training (HIT) to build his championship physique.[4] This contrasted with standard bodybuilding programs of the time (promoted by Arnold Schwarzenegger and the like, so plenty of people took notice).[5]

If you're feeling cynical, you could argue that because all these men were on huge doses of steroids and other performance-enhancing drugs, their success with a method can't be seen as proof it works. And that's a fair

1   G Nuckols (2017) *Bulgarian Manual* [online], available at
     www.strongerbyscience.com/bulgarian-manual
2   P Tsatsouline (2003) *The Naked Warrior*. Saint Paul, MN: Dragon Door
     Publications.
3   P Tsatsouline and D John (2011) *Easy Strength*. Saint Paul, MN:
     Dragon Door Publications.
4   https://blog.dynutrition.com/blood-and-guts-hit-system
5   A Schwarzenegger (2012) *The Encylopaedia of Modern Bodybuilding*.
     New York: Simon and Schuster.

point, but it's at least worth noting that these options are out there.

But the number of choices and theories about training frequency is exactly what's made the topic so muddled. There are a lot of different approaches because people historically relied on anecdotes over science. Because they weren't taking a rigorous approach to their training, they didn't make sure they held other variables (like volume, intensity and exercise selection) constant. This meant that any studies were moderately useful at best.

That was until 2012, when the Norwegian Frequency Project was carried out.[6] This study took a group of trained powerlifters and split them in two. To give you an idea of the experience levels of the trainees, they were all between eighteen and twenty-five years old, squatting 125–205 kg, benching 85–165 kg and deadlifting between 155–245 kg. These are not huge numbers at the lower end, but they were certainly not novices. And that's important because what works for a novice isn't guaranteed to work for anyone more experienced.

One half of the group trained three days a week, the other trained six days a week. Everything else remained the same: same exercises, same routine, same total volume and intensity. After fifteen weeks of training, the

---

6   https://mennohenselmans.com/norwegian-frequency-project-stats

results were astounding. The group training six times a week gained twice as much strength as those on the three-day routine (an average gain of 10% vs 5%).

This study was significant because it was the first time that a group of trained individuals had been put through their paces in a rigorous manner. The only thing that was different between the two groups was the frequency of their sessions. Simply by training twice as frequently, one group was able to get twice the gains of the other. The question, of course, is why was this the case?

The existing body of research suggests some different reasons as to why training more frequently is great for boosting your gains.[7] One potential factor is that the muscle-building effect of training (ie its impact on muscle protein synthesis) peaks in the first twenty-four hours after training, tapering off until seventy-two hours after the session. By training more frequently, you can keep the fires burning for longer and build more muscle, which equates to more strength potential in the long run.

Another factor is that by dividing up your sessions, you're less tired at the start of each session. The less tired you are, the better your technique will be. And as we already know that strength has a skill component,

---

7   https://mennohenselmans.com/norwegian-frequency-project-stats

this will help you get stronger over the course of several weeks.

Finally, the more often you do something, the easier it gets. The more often you lift a weight that's decently challenging, the easier you'll find it. An interesting point to note here is that upper body exercises benefit more from high-frequency training than lower body ones.

Training more frequently will probably allow you to increase your training volume, not just match it. For instance, if you only bench press twice a week for five sets, that's ten sets total. Training bench four days a week for three sets per session is twelve sets total – more overall volume. We'll discuss this in more detail in the section about training volume, but it seems as if more volume (that you can recover from) = more gains. And if more frequency = better gains with equal volume, it's possible that more volume + more frequency = even better gains.

Overall, the results are clear – training more frequently is better than training less frequently (at least for strength). But of course, we always have to temper the findings of research with reality. Training six times a week may be more effective than training three times a week, but if you don't have time to get to the gym that often, what good does that information do you?

That's the lie of the land when it comes to training frequency for strength development and muscle gain.

Useful, but not the final answer. Of course, studies are good for showing us how people will respond on average. You can guarantee that there are outliers in any study. Some will do exceptionally well, some will do poorly and others will get normal results. It's the same in your training, and in your life. Perhaps high-frequency is the key to unlocking more gains than ever before, or maybe not.

When creating programs, I like to see trainees in the gym three to five times a week. In my opinion, that's a solid middle ground that fits with their lives, gets most of the results associated with frequent training and leaves them well set to succeed moving forward.

Another reason why I like higher frequency programs (within reason) is that they help to keep trainees on track. Think about it: if you're training first thing in the morning four or five days a week, that sets the tone for your whole day. It can help you make better food choices, get you to bed at a reasonable time, give you more energy after the session... the list goes on.

Doing something regularly is good for making it into a habit. Training once or twice a week looks easy on paper, but it's also simple to discount the role of training in your life. You could end up shunting it around your calendar, never giving it the attention it needs.

Three days a week can be the perfect choice for someone who's busy, but still looking to make serious progress.

With intelligent planning, you can achieve fantastic results on a three-day setup.

Individual adaptation is a given once you've gained a little experience. It can be beneficial to play around with some of the variables in your training to see how it affects your results, but I discourage beginners from doing so as it's easy to lose sight of the bigger picture.

Changing how frequently you train can be a useful tool to stimulate new progress if you've been stuck at a plateau. Going from five days a week to three can allow you to push harder during each session, which in turn can get you out of your rut and back on track.

Frequency is just one of the variables that matter when it comes to training. Next, let's take a look at the role of volume.

Training volume

Principle 1: training volume is best measured by looking at the number of hard sets you're doing (hard = pushing yourself to near the point of failure).

Principle 2: building some flexibility into your programming is a good way to manage recovery. You can do this by having minimum and maximum sets/reps to aim for in a given workout, and by progressively adding volume over time.

Training volume is another factor that's proved contentious among experts in the past. For most people, volume, intensity and frequency are all roughly related to one another. The higher your volume, the lower your intensity and frequency will be, and vice versa. You can't maintain high-volume, high-intensity and high-frequency routines for any length of time as a natural trainee. It's different if you're fuelled by anabolic steroids, of course, but that's a topic for another day!

Certain routines do attempt to balance relatively high levels of volume, frequency and intensity. One such program is the Smolov Squat Routine.[8] It's notoriously difficult, but trainees report good results if they manage to push through.

At the high end of the volume spectrum is German Volume Training (GVT),[9] which is a fancy name for what's a pretty simple system (simple to understand, not simple to do). Basically, it's ten sets of ten for various exercises, short rest periods and a decently challenging load.

On the low-volume end of the spectrum, we return once again to HIT proponents like Dorian Yates and Mike Mentzer. These men preferred to do just a couple of sets per exercise, but to do them to failure. And in

---

8   www.smolovjr.com/smolov-squat-routine
9   www.bodybuilding.com/content/german-volume-training
     -programs.html

doing so, they got results that were just as good as any, without spending a lot of time in the gym.

We'll deal with training intensity in the next section, but for now, it's important to note that training hard (ie using heavy weights) takes a significant toll on your body. It's a trade-off between the more acute stress of doing a few all-out sets and doing more, but not as hard.

No discussion of volume would be complete without referring to the sets and reps used in your programming. And yes, this is the easiest way to quantify training volume. But volume also has to be considered over a longer period of time. As we saw in the previous section on frequency, spreading training volume out over the course of a week still gets you the results you're after.

If you've done any research into the topic of getting bigger and stronger, you've probably heard something like:

- Do sets of one to five reps for strength

- Do sets of eight to twelve reps for building muscle

- Do sets of fifteen to twenty reps for endurance

And as for sets? Here are some pretty common recommendations:

- Three to five sets of three to five reps for strength

- Four to five sets of eight to twelve reps for size

- Four to five sets of fifteen to twenty reps for endurance

And honestly, these recommendations are fine. If you follow them, they work pretty well, but it's important to note that just because they work well doesn't mean that something else won't work better.

There are inherent drawbacks to lifting heavy weights all the time, or lifting light weights every workout. Over the course of weeks and months, your body can stop adapting to the stress you're placing on it to the point where it stops having any noticeable effect on you. And even leaving aside the fact that your body adapts to whatever stress you put on it, it's important to note that volume adds up over the course of weeks and months. Following a high-volume routine can be a great way to push past your limits for a month or two, but if you're continuously doing more than you can recover from, you'll soon pay the price for your folly.

It's not as straightforward as simply saying, 'Do x sets of this exercise four times a week and call it a day.' In practice, it's much more complicated. There are essentially two schools of thought when it comes to programming volume:

- Do as little as possible to achieve the desired result – the minimum effective dose

- Do as much as you can recover from, as this will allow you to get all the gains you possibly can

In my opinion, aiming for either of these extremes will set you up for failure. Yes, it's good to be efficient. We're all living busy lives and don't want to waste time eking out another 2% on a maximum lift when we could be using it for something else. Yes, it's good to push ourselves and squeeze more results out of our routine if we can. Within reason, doing more gets us more (assuming we can recover and continue to progress).

That said, training is not an exact science. We are not machines. There is no handbook to give us the precise sets, reps, exercises and routine to take us from zero to absolute unit. It's impossible to know if five reps is all we need to get stronger (or five sets, or three workouts in the week). Likewise, knowing we can theoretically recover from x amount of volume per week is all well and good, but does it have any bearing on reality? If all it takes to derail your program is a few bad nights' sleep, a stressful week at work or a case of indigestion, your program needs to change.

Personally, I like to work a bit of flexibility into my programs. Creating something that you can stick with for the long haul is more important than creating the perfect program you can't do. One simple way I work in flexibility is by setting minimum and maximum volume targets for exercises and workouts. While the exact methods I use when writing a program depend on the needs of the individual, this is one I commonly employ.

For example, I could create a program that has you doing three to five sets of six to eight reps on bench twice a week. On the days when you're feeling great, you have the option to hit another few sets, or even work up to a new maximum on occasion. On the days when you're dragging and can barely muster up the energy to hit your minimums, that's all you have to do.

All training puts stress on your body. The goal is to push yourself into the red, but not so far that you can't get yourself back out. Having the option to adapt your volume from workout to workout helps you to manage recovery more effectively, which sets you up for success in the long term. Of course, managing volume is something that you have to take a longer perspective on – it's not simply a matter of seeing what looks good on paper for a given week.

When it comes to measuring volume, there are a few approaches people like to use. One common method is to measure volume in terms of sets × reps × weight used. That's fine in certain situations, but there are several problems with this approach.

For a start, if more volume = more gains, it would be easy to assume that inherently heavier exercises would be better for driving gains. Applying that logic, you could assume that leg pressing is better than squatting simply because you can use more weight on it, or that machine bench pressing is superior to bench pressing, but using more weight isn't always the answer. Additionally, assuming that more volume = more gains (when volume is measured as sets × reps × weight used) would lead you to use less weight than you're capable of. For instance, someone with a bench press maximum of 200 kg can probably do five reps with 180 kg, ten reps with 140 kg and twenty+ reps with 100 kg. (These are all just rough numbers – I'll explain how I calculated them in the next section.)

Let's calculate the total volume at each weight:

- 200 kg × one rep = 200 kg volume

- 180 kg × five reps = 900 kg volume

- 140 kg × ten reps = 1,400 kg volume

- 100 kg × twenty reps = 2,000 kg volume

Based purely on this formula, it appears as if doing less weight for more reps is up to ten times better than simply focusing on your maximum. While I'm a big advocate of avoiding constant strength tests and laying a foundation of strength in higher rep ranges, I know that plenty of people do fine with lower rep workouts. And certainly, doing nothing but twenty rep sets isn't the shortcut to making easy gains.

We'll touch on this topic more in the next section regarding intensity, but for now, let's reiterate that sets × reps × weight is *not* the best measure of volume. In my experience, it's far easier to keep track of the number of hard sets you're doing in your routine. Whether those sets are ten reps, fifteen reps, five reps or three reps matters less than simply getting in there and pushing yourself hard to improve. Hard sets of eight to twelve reps are easier to recover from than sets of three to five reps (due to nervous system fatigue etc), but they all have their place in a well-structured routine.

I like to see people work in a variety of rep ranges for different exercises. Most of the time, we'll be dealing with sets in the 70%+ intensity range (more on that soon), but lighter training has a place in the system too.

Properly managing volume is a balancing act. Too little, and you'll see no results. Too much, and you'll be unable to recover. With experience, staying between the lines gets easier. Building an element of volume management into your program is a good way to do this.

Next, we turn our attention to how much weight you actually lift.

Intensity

Principle 1: spend the majority of your training time working with weights in the 70–90% range, occasionally going lower or higher depending on your needs.

Principle 2: making progress (and giving each set your best effort) is the name of the game.

We can think about intensity in a few different ways. Most people think it refers to how much effort we're putting into our training. But what constitutes effort and how do we measure it? Without a clear answer to these questions, we default to simple benchmarks, like:

- How red our face gets

- How loudly we grunt

- How hard we slam our weights back in the rack after a heavy set

It's easy to equate training hard with being loud, aggressive and visible. Fitness bros on YouTube and Instagram have big audiences for a reason. The reality is that these guys have to put on a show to keep their audience entertained. In putting on a hyped-up persona for the camera, they lead people to believe that this kind of approach is necessary to make serious gains.

Of course, superficial measures are a poor proxy for how hard you're truly training. It's easy to fake intensity by screaming out every set like it's your last; it's a lot harder to actually get stronger over time, without the bullshit.

I like to see trainees putting in a good shift in the gym. I've nothing against people getting hyped up before a maximum set or having a training partner spur them on to get a few more reps when it's safe to do so; what I'm not on board with is people pushing themselves beyond the point of safety on a regular basis. Additionally, I'm not a massive fan of getting hyped up every workout for all sets.

My perspective is this: if you can't hit a certain lift without three cups of coffee, your favourite heavy metal music playing and your lucky shoes, then can you honestly say you're strong enough to do it? Don't get me wrong – I love a good cup of coffee. And music that gets you in the zone is a big boost for anyone. But if you're reliant on these things? If you need to have your eyes popping out of your head to hit your next set? You're fighting a losing battle.

Now that we've talked about the more informal definition of intensity, let's talk about the scientific definition. Intensity is the amount of weight you're using relative to the maximum weight you could use. For instance, if your maximum bench press is 200 kg, then benching

STRONGER MIND, STRONGER BODY, STRONGER LIFE

180 kg is 90% intensity (as 180 is 90% of 200). To run through the numbers quickly:

- 200 kg = 100% intensity
- 180 kg = 90% intensity
- 160 kg = 80% intensity
- 140 kg = 70% intensity
- 120 kg = 60% intensity
- 100 kg = 50% intensity

The higher your intensity, the less overall volume you're going to be able to handle. You can get a lot more reps in with 50% of your maximum weight than with 90% of it, but as sets × reps × weight is not the best measure of volume, it's more advantageous to count the number of hard sets you're doing in a given workout/week.

In my experience, I've found that we rarely know how far we can truly push ourselves. Our brain wants to give in long before our body needs the break. David Goggins (Navy SEAL, ultra-endurance runner and all around physical badass) coined the 40% Rule.[10] Simply put, he believes that when you feel like giving up, you're only 40% done. While we can argue about the

---

10 D Goggins (2018) *Can't Hurt Me: Master your mind and defy the odds.* New York: Lioncrest Publishing.

exact percentages, the fact remains that we can do more than we think we can. The harder we push ourselves (within reason), the better the results we'll get.

I like to have trainees push to the point of either momentary muscular failure (where safe), or only being able to do one to two more reps. I'm talking 'gun to your head' levels of exertion – get to the point where you could only do another rep or two if your life was on the line, and you'll be pushing yourself hard enough to make serious gains.

I'd like to round off this section by giving you a handy formula to calculate the estimated number of reps you should be able to get with a given percentage of your one-rep maximum. For every 3% you take off your one-rep maximum, you can do one more rep. That means you could do:

- One rep with 100% of your maximum

- Five reps with 88% of your maximum

- Ten reps with 72% of your maximum

I like to see trainees hit most of their sets in the 5–12 rep range, working close to the point of failure (or up to the point of momentary muscular failure in some cases). Spending most of your training time in the 70–90% range is best for developing a solid combination of strength and size.

Of course, it's good to round out your training with some higher rep and lower rep sets too. If you're aiming to set a new maximum, it can be helpful to ease into it by working with heavier weights for a week or two beforehand. And working with slightly lighter weights can be good to get more volume without adding too much stress to your joints.

The decision as to how heavy to go on a particular exercise depends on the movement itself. For instance, it's relatively easy (and safe) to lift heavier weights on a compound movement like a bench press or squat. It's harder to do it safely with a single-joint exercise like a curl as there's more potential for injury.

That same truth applies to how hard you should push yourself on a particular exercise. Don't push yourself past the point of form breakdown on a bigger exercise like a deadlift as there's too much risk of injury. On the other hand, you can push yourself a little more on isolation exercises (within reason) as they pose less of a danger.

Let's round off this chapter on programming by talking about something pretty simple, but often overlooked.

Rest periods

Principle: the more out of shape you are, the more rest you'll need to recover from a particular set.

We don't need to spend much time on this section, as the facts around rest periods are pretty well defined. A lot of popular beginner workouts recommend that trainees take as much rest between sets as they need to feel totally recovered. For instance, take Starting Strength.[11]

For those of you who don't know, Starting Strength is a popular novice routine. The program is simple:

- Work out three days a week

- Squat three days a week (three sets of five)

- Alternate between bench press and overhead press (three sets of five)

- Deadlift once a week (one set of five)

- Power clean twice a week (five sets of three)

- Add weight every time you do these

Among other recommendations, the program prescribes rest periods of three to five minutes, or even longer as you get towards the end of the program.

As the name suggests, this is a program best left to *novices*. Novices are capable of adding weight every workout as they're getting better at doing the exercise (technique-wise, on a neurological basis). I'm torn in

---

11   https://startingstrength.com

my analysis of a program like this. On one hand, it's good for getting novices from weak to decently strong in as fast a period of time as possible. But on the other hand, I don't simply define strength as the maximum weight a trainee can lift for a few reps. Lifting heavier weights is all well and good, but if you require five-minute rest periods between efforts, what good is that to you in real life?

I'm a firm believer that your training should develop multiple qualities at once. Getting bigger and stronger is good, but also improve your cardiovascular fitness at the same time. I like to see trainees pushing themselves to maintain a decent level of output all throughout their session. I don't look for them to have heart rates of 150 beats per minute, but it's good if they're still a little out of breath when commencing their next set.

On a physiological level, one of the principal substances responsible for power output (ie the mechanism used to lift the weight you're working with) is adenosine triphosphate (ATP). ATP recovery is linked to how much rest you take between sets. According to the most trusted research,[12] here's the timeline for ATP recovery:

12 J S Baker, M C McCormick and R A Robergs (2010)
    'Interaction among Skeletal Muscle Metabolic Energy
    Systems during Intense Exercise', J Nutr Metab 2010: 905612,
    www.ncbi.nlm.nih.gov/pmc/articles/PMC3005844

Rest period	Amount of ATP replenished
Thirty seconds	50%
One minute	75%
Ninety seconds	87%
Two minutes	93%
Two-and-a-half minutes	97%
Three minutes	98.50%

These are general guidelines – your specific recovery times may differ, but the point remains that after ninety seconds, your ATP will have recovered by almost 90%. This means that you'll be well able to move on and complete your next set, provided you're not going for a new maximum or something similar.

I like to see trainees take between one to two minutes of rest between sets, depending on how much weight they're using. At that rate, they recover enough to give a good effort in their next set while minimising their downtime in the gym.

The time you spend resting between sets can add up quickly if you're not vigilant. Using a basic stopwatch app on your phone (and sticking to it) is all you need to do to combat this. Don't sit on a bench or take up equipment in the gym while you scroll through social media on your phone under the guise of taking a rest period. You're not in the gym to waste time. You have other commitments in your life – every second wasted on bullshit is another second you'll never get back.

To save even more time in the gym, I often recommend super-setting complementary exercises. For instance, let's say you have five sets of bench press and five sets of barbell rows to get through. The typical way to do this workout would be to do all your sets of bench press first, then move on to rows.

Straight sets:

- Bench press – set one
- Rest two minutes
- Bench press – set two
- Rest two minutes
- Bench press – set three
- Rest two minutes
- Bench press – set four
- Rest two minutes
- Bench press – set five
- Move on to barbell rows

That's fine, but there's a lot of dead time in there.

Rather than doing a set of bench press, resting for two minutes, doing another set, then resting again, you could super-set – alternate between sets of each exercise, cutting the rest periods in half for the same overall effect. It would look like this:

- Bench press – set one
- Rest one minute
- Barbell rows – set one
- Rest one minute
- Bench press – set two
- Rest one minute
- Barbell rows – set two
- Rest one minute
- Bench press – set three
- Rest one minute
- Barbell rows – set three
- Rest one minute
- Bench press – set four
- Rest one minute
- Barbell rows – set four
- Rest one minute
- Bench press – set five
- Rest one minute
- Barbell rows – set five
- Rest one minute

In this example, you've completed twice the amount of work (ten sets vs five) with the same amount of rest. You'll be more efficient in the gym, taxing your conditioning more and building your work capacity – which is of great benefit in the long term. Good all round.

There are other techniques you can employ. You've probably come across circuit training before (where you stack multiple different exercises together without a rest, then take a break at the end). When it's designed intelligently, this can be a great tool in your programming arsenal, but it's important to avoid a setup that requires you to tie up several pieces of equipment at once or has you using much less weight than you could be.

To sum it up: shorter rest periods are better than excessively long ones. You can still build plenty of strength resting just one to two minutes between sets, and the additional benefits of improving your cardiovascular fitness make any potential drop-off in the weight you're using worth it.

10
Nutrition Is Key

Now that we've got a firm grasp on the principles of effective training, it's time to turn our attention to the second vital piece of building a strong body: nutrition. As the old saying goes, you are what you eat. This isn't a metaphor; it's literal. The foods you eat will influence the man you become, acting as the building blocks you use to transform your body and life as you walk along the path.

Much like training, nutrition is a subject many people overcomplicate. In reality, all you need to succeed is to understand and apply the basics. That's true of most things in life, but it's particularly true when it comes to building a strong body, so in this chapter, we'll cover the fundamentals of effective nutrition.

Specifically, here's what we'll talk about:

- The most basic terms you'll hear about diet and what they mean, including the essential nutrients your body needs for optimal health and performance

- The fundamental eating style you need to be familiar with

- My hard and fast rules for effective nutrition – just follow these principles and you'll be fine

Eating in accordance with your goals is critical to transforming your body. Without giving your body the materials it needs to recover and grow stronger, you'll be fighting an uphill battle all the way. Don't make walking the path more difficult than it needs to be. Use the knowledge in this chapter as an asset that drives you forward towards your goals.

The basic nutrition terms – micros, macros and more

It's easy to get confused when you're confronted with a new diet plan. Faced with jargon that looks like it'd be more at home in a chemistry textbook, a nutrient timing protocol more complicated than a rocket launch and a supplement list longer than your arm, you may be put off and think that it's not worth the time to master this area of physical transformation. And to be honest? I'm right there with you.

I don't believe in making this process more complicated than it needs to be. But once you understand the fundamental terms, what they mean and – most importantly – how you can use that information, you're good to go. In this section, we're going to cover the most important terms to understand for what's to come.

Calorie. There's a formal scientific definition of calorie and then there's the one we care about. To keep things relevant, think of it this way: a calorie is a unit of energy. The more calories something has, the more energy it will give people. Note that this energy isn't necessarily the kind that will have you hopping off the walls with newfound vigour. Feeling energetic and taking in more calories are not always linked.

Macronutrient. A macronutrient (macro) is a substance (nutrient) that your body needs in large quantities to function. The three primary macros are *fats, carbohydrates* and *proteins*. Pretty much all foods will have some amount of each of these macros in them – all that changes is the ratio of each substance in different foods.

For instance, a chicken breast has far more protein in it than a carrot. Peanuts have more fat in them than a lean cut of steak. Oatmeal has more carbohydrates than celery. Learning to balance your diet with foods that give you ample amounts of each macro is the key to nutritional success.

Micronutrients. These are substances that your body needs, but not in the same quantities as macros.

Micronutrients (micros) are found in all the same foods you'll get your macros from and play a valuable role in regulating your metabolism, hormones and health in general. In simple terms, we're talking about vitamins and minerals when we reference micros. We'll discuss these in more detail in the section about supplements in Chapter 11.

Fats. Fat is one of the primary macros. It's the most energy-dense of the bunch at 9 calories per gram, but fats aren't something to be afraid of. On the contrary, they're an important part of any healthy diet, playing a role in brain function, hormonal health and more. Depending on the particular diet you follow, fats could account for anything from 15–80% of your daily calorie intake.

There is a distinction between healthy and unhealthy fats. The general rule of thumb is that natural fat sources are fine (which means that saturated fat is not a problem), whereas lab-created trans fats are not.

Carbohydrates (carbs) have been demonised in recent times. Once they were thought of as a staple of any healthy diet, but some newer diets see them omitted almost completely.

For most people, carbs serve a purpose. They play a vital role in energy production, are cheap to buy and are a good way to get in extra calories for those looking to build muscle.

Carbs can be simple or complex. For instance, sugary foods are high in simple carbs – they hit your bloodstream quickly, but see you crash soon after. In contrast, complex carbs (eg oatmeal or vegetables) take longer to digest, giving you stable energy over a longer period of time. Carbs come in at 4 calories per gram, which means you need to eat more of them to get the same energy you'd get from fat.

Protein is probably the most significant macro for muscle growth. At 4 calories per gram, it's as energy-dense as carbs. Protein is made up of amino acids (substances your body uses to repair muscle tissue, grow and keep you healthy). Without adequate levels of protein intake, you'll never achieve optimal results.

The amount that is adequate has been the subject of much debate over the years. Some people recommend eating as much as you can (eg 300–400 g a day), whereas other diets could have you eating 100 g per day. Results vary depending on personal makeup. Personally, I like to see people strike a happy medium.

Now that we're clear on these six basic terms, let's move on and talk about the only eating style to get a solid handle on your nutrition moving forward.

The fundamental eating style

When you do a little research online about different diets, you'll probably see the same protocols coming up again and again:

- Vegetarian
- Vegan
- Carnivore
- Paleo
- Keto
- Atkins

Many different diets, all claiming to offer health benefits that none of the others can provide. All say that their way is the best way, and that choosing anything else is a huge waste of time. With so much conflicting information out there, it's easy to see why you'd get confused. But believe me, you don't need to be.

Fundamentally, the most important part of any diet is figuring out if it will help you meet your goals. And that comes down to whether it gives you enough of the stuff you need (and minimises the rest). By far the best approach I've come across is flexible dieting. You might have seen this referenced as 'if it fits your macros' (IIFYM). Essentially, this style of eating transcends the other options.

Rather than stipulating that you have to eat certain foods or consume exact ratios of certain macros, IIFYM says that all that really matters is giving your body enough of what it needs (then leaving the rest up to you). Let's explain this with an example. Say you want to enrol on my online coaching program. Your goal is to lose weight, as at 200 lb, you're 30 lb heavier than you'd like to be. After asking you some questions and plugging your details into a certain formula (which we'll cover later on), I then tell you that your daily calorie target is 2,000. Consuming this number, assuming we've calculated it correctly based on your lifestyle and exercise routine, will see you losing weight steadily. We then take that daily calorie goal and figure out the correct amounts of each macro.

Here's how each macro stacks up against each other:

- Carbs = 4 calories per gram

- Protein = 4 calories per gram

- Fat = 9 calories per gram

Once we have these figures in mind, we then move on and establish baseline amounts of each macronutrient to include in your diet. Based on my experience, I've seen that good target minimums (for most people) are:

- Protein: 0.7 g per lb of bodyweight

- Carbs = no set minimum (although I rarely prescribe less than 0.5 g per lb of bodyweight)

- Fat = 0.35 g per lb of bodyweight

If you weigh 200 lbs, here's what your minimums of each look like:

- Protein = 200 lbs × 0.7 = 140 g

- Carbs = 200 lbs × 0.5 = 100 g

- Fat = 200 lbs × 0.35 = 70 g

Bearing in mind your daily target of 2,000 calories, let's see how much wiggle room you have left to play around with:

- Protein = 140 g × 4 calories per gram = 560 calories

- Carbs = 100 g × 4 calories per gram = 400 calories

- Fat = 70 g × 9 calories per gram = 630 calories

- 560 + 400 + 630 = 1,590 calories

- 2,000 − 1,590 = 410 calories left over

On an IIFYM protocol, you're free to allocate these calories wherever you like. More fats, more carbs or more protein – the point is you can adjust based on personal preference and find out what works best for you. As long as you hit your minimums of each macro and total calories for the day, you're good to go.

While an IIFYM will give you a fixed number to aim for, it doesn't tell you exactly what foods you need to eat. And there's where it really shines. Having flexibility in your diet allows you to pick and choose to include foods you enjoy, sprinkling them in wherever they fit. If you hate eating chicken, you don't need to eat it – just pick something else as your protein source. Likewise, if you want to eat some chocolate or a pizza, you don't need to deprive yourself. If it fits into your daily numbers, you're good to go. Note that there is a difference between eating for optimal health and performance and eating just for body recomposition (which is what IIFYM is for), but we'll touch on that later.

The particular macro split that works best for you will be different to what works for me. For instance, some people respond well to carbs, whereas others do best with almost zero carbs. Some perform well on high-fat diets, while others find a moderate approach more effective. Personal experimentation is key. That's how you figure out what strategy fits your lifestyle and unique physiological makeup.

IIFYM/flexible dieting is the best approach to take for building a strong body. This is because you can seamlessly choose to follow any other eating style while also following this one. There's nothing to say that you can't be vegan following this protocol – your pool of potential foods will be more limited, but you can do it.

Of course, there are some ways to do this that are better than others. In the next section, I'll detail some different rules to consider if you want to use this protocol effectively. But when it boils down to it, IIFYM is the simplest, most effective approach you can take. It gives you the freedom you need to avoid going crazy on some convoluted diet, and most importantly? It's sustainable for the long haul. And as you walk the path of the strong, having a solid, flexible diet plan could be the difference between success and failure.

To get started with this approach, please visit www .gavinmeenan.com/macros. There, you'll be able to get a full breakdown of your macros using the formula we touched on earlier, as well as some sample foods and meals to help you hit your goals.

Now that we've introduced IIFYM as an eating style, let's talk about how you can make it work for you.

My rules for effective nutrition

IIFYM sounds great on paper. Eat whatever you want, whenever you want. Don't worry about the fine details – just hit your numbers and you'll be fine. But sadly, it's not quite as simple as that in practice.

While the flexibility offered by IIFYM is a huge plus for pretty much all the clients I've prescribed it for, I've also found that giving them a list of general rules to abide by is helpful. These rules give them a framework that guides them to make better decisions, leading to better outcomes: more energy, more robust health, increased performance in the gym and more.

Rule 1: Food quality matters

I've seen too many people who have used the excuse of 'But it fits my macros!' to justify feasting on junk food, binge drinking beer and partaking in other questionable activities. And on one hand, they're right. For the purposes of improving your body composition, all that truly matters is getting your macros in. Your body doesn't necessarily view the carbs that come in the form of a chocolate bar any differently to those that come from oatmeal once they're broken down into their base form. But even if you can eat pizza for every meal and lose weight, it doesn't take a genius to figure out this is a bad idea.

Food quality matters. If the majority of your food choices are shit, you will feel like shit. IIFYM offers you the freedom to sprinkle in foods that you enjoy, even if they aren't 100% healthy, but if your diet is all sprinkles and no substance, you're in for a bad time.

I encourage my clients to eat in accordance with the 80/20 or 90/10 principle,[1] depending on their starting point and goals. I don't mind seeing 10–20% of their daily calories coming from less-than-healthy options, but anything more than that? The negative side effects of eating junk far outweigh whatever benefits they think they're getting.

---

1   R Koch (2011) *The 80/20 Principle*. New York: Nicholas Brealey Publishing.

No one's saying you can't have the occasional off day, but again, this is about consistency. Keep the days you spend off the wagon to a minimum and you'll keep making progress. But if you lose sight of your goal, you could end up trapped by poor eating habits that will require a lot of effort to break.

Principle 2: Meal timing is up to you

Meal timing is the subject of much debate in the online fitness space. And I'm here to tell you that unless you're a high-level athlete or looking to squeeze out the last 5–10% of your gains, don't worry too much about it.

Once again, I like to see people start from somewhere reasonable, then experiment to see what works best for them. For instance, you'll probably find that eating some kind of fast-acting carb (eg a banana) before your gym session gives you a quick energy boost. But maybe you'd perform even better if you ate a little protein along with this. Or if you ate nothing at all. Or if you ate a little closer or further away from your start time.

The point here is that worrying too much about meal timing is a fool's game. The specifics of the subject are too nuanced to be worth the effort you need to figure it out. Instead, focus on getting a handle on the basics.

See how your pre-workout meal affects you. Do you do best with a little food in your stomach? Or do you prefer to work out after fasting? See how you feel about eating late at night. Does it help you sleep better? Or are you up for hours with heartburn and indigestion? Play around with your coffee intake. Do you like it an hour before the gym? Or do you prefer not to be too stimulated heading in?

It's all a matter of personal experimentation. What works best for you is unique to your makeup – but don't stress about meal timing too much. For the average guy looking to build a stronger body, there's no need. Just eat well, train hard and let the rest fall into place.

Principle 3: A little is better than a lot

When it comes to choosing foods that meet their macros, many people go overboard and use things like Pop Tarts as a staple source of carbs or greasy fast food for a quick hit of protein. As I've said before, there's nothing wrong with including a small amount of these foods in your diet, but moderation is key.

You're better off consuming a little of something on a regular basis rather than engaging in less frequent but much more damaging binges. I would prefer to see someone eat ice cream every night than take a weekend off every month to eat and drink themselves into oblivion.

Your mileage may vary, of course. Maybe you find it easier to completely abstain from your vices, then go crazy every once in a while. But if you're like most people, you'll probably find moderation is a better, more sustainable approach. When you know you can have a little bit of what you fancy anytime you want it (provided you stay within your numbers), you'll have a much easier time staying disciplined with your diet. Bear this principle in mind when you're using an IIFYM approach and you'll set yourself up for success.

Principle 4: Stay hydrated

Staying hydrated is one of the biggest things you need to focus on for health and performance. Two simple rules of thumb:

- Drink at least 2 litres of water per day (good for general health). That amount will increase if you live somewhere hot or are very active.

- Think carefully before ingesting too many liquid calories. They're a great asset for someone bulking – not so much if you're trying to lose weight.

That's it. Regardless of the diet plan you follow, stay hydrated. The health benefits of doing so are too numerous to mention, and besides, do you really need to be told that drinking water is good for you? Just do it!

Principle 5: Don't fall prey to the fear

You don't have to look too far to see examples of nutritional fear mongering. Whether it's a story about red meat causing cancer, animal products killing the planet, artificial sweeteners poisoning you or sugar being the downfall of Western civilisation, there's a headline out there to grab your attention and stimulate your fear response. I'm not saying whether any of these statements are true or false. All I'm saying is don't fall prey to the fear.

Once you've got a good grasp of how to eat well, you don't need to worry too much about what the headlines are screaming at you. Everything in moderation. Don't eat like an idiot; be reasonable and you'll do just fine.

Basic tips anyone can follow to eat better:

- Eat as few processed foods as possible
- Enjoy alcohol, sugar and refined carbs only occasionally
- Try to eat a decent mix of foods – don't eat the same four meals every day
- If something makes you tired, sick or unhappy, cut it out
- If something makes you feel better, eat more of it
- Get your fruits and vegetables in
- Don't treat food like it's a reward all the time

That's it. Follow these rules and your nutrition is 80% optimised. Everything else is just window dressing.

CASE STUDY: KEVIN THE BODYBUILDER

Kevin had a physique that most guys would kill for, but it still wasn't enough to make him happy. An avid bodybuilder since his days spent pumping out rep after rep on a rickety old bench in his childhood bedroom, Kevin had gone on to achieve great things. He routinely competed in top amateur bodybuilding competitions all around the world, often ranking well and sometimes winning.

After several years at the top, Kevin was ready to come down. The only problem was that he had forgotten how to get off this ride. Multiple six-month cycles of meticulous contest prep had destroyed Kevin's relationship with food. Everything that appeared on his plate was judged by the numbers. If it didn't fit his plan perfectly, he wouldn't eat it.

Additionally, his gruelling pre-competition workouts had left him sick of the gym. He often ended up taking a month off in between events because he couldn't stomach the idea of walking through those doors again.

When I met Kevin, he had finished competing as an amateur bodybuilder, but still wanted to keep training and eating well for the numerous health benefits of doing so. Kevin's main problem wasn't a lack of knowledge. In fact, he was a guy who could have easily made a living as a personal trainer if he desired. No, his problem was between his ears.

In my work with Kevin, I helped him to rediscover a couple of key principles his obsessive paradigm had rendered invisible through years of conditioning:

- Having 6% body fat is not that much better than 8%, or 10% or 12%
- Eating well doesn't mean eating purely by the numbers at all times
- If you're not enjoying your workouts, you're doing something wrong

Once we had decided on the principles Kevin would use to guide his training and dietary choices moving forward, we worked together to develop a regime that met his needs. I deliberately encouraged Kevin to mix some unhealthy foods into his diet. Was this *technically* the most effective approach? No, but for someone who had almost developed an eating disorder through years of obsession, it was necessary.

I'm happy to report that Kevin is firmly on track with his training and diet these days. While he's no longer a client, he keeps in touch with me. He works out three to four times a week, eats well and does his best to keep his stress low. But if life throws him a curveball, he doesn't worry about it. Shit happens – all you can do is keep moving forward.

11

Supplements and Steroids

Supplements

If you've been in the fitness space for any length of time, then you'll know that there are a lot of poor-quality supplements out there – 80% hype, 15% placebo, 5% actual effect is the standard formula. In this section, I'll give you a quick-fire rundown of the best supplements you can take – the ones that give you the best bang for your buck. The products I introduce to you here may be familiar, but I'd bet there are a few you're not taking regularly for one reason or another.

Creatine

Creatine is a molecule that is used by your body to create energy when you place your muscles under stress (ie when you're pushing out the last few reps of an exercise). Logically enough, more creatine in your system means that your body will be able to create more energy, allowing you to lift heavier weights and/or do more reps on any given exercise.

While creatine is found in food such as meat, fish and eggs, it's much more efficient to get it via supplementation. Supplementing with creatine achieves two main things:

1. It increases your power output

2. It helps you retain more water (which makes you heavier)

The primary benefit of creatine is that it increases your power output. After a week or so of taking it, you'll see a noticeable increase in strength-related performance. The secondary effect of creatine is that you'll gain weight fairly quickly after you start taking it (2–3 kg). This is nothing to worry about: it's just water weight, and you'll lose it again if you stop taking creatine for an extended period of time.

Creatine is dirt-cheap. You can get a 250 g bag of creatine monohydrate (this is the type you should take) for under €10 on any of the major supplement sites – www.myprotein.com, www.bulkpowders.co.uk etc – or for a little more in a physical store.

To take creatine, simply measure 5–10 g of it into at least 500 ml of water using the scoop provided, then drink it down. I recommend starting with 5 g, only scaling up to 10 g if you're not seeing the benefits within a week or two.

You can take creatine indefinitely – there's no need to cycle off it. You can take it any time of the day – morning or night, it's all the same (and don't worry about taking it pre- or post-workout, as it makes no difference).

One thing you'll want to do is drink plenty of water when you're taking creatine. A lot of people notice some stomach issues (cramps, nausea etc) if they don't stay hydrated while taking this. If you experience consistent issues, try spreading your intake out across the day (eg half a dose in the morning, half in the evening).

Whey protein

Whey is one of two proteins that naturally occur in milk (the other being casein, which is another fine choice). If you've ever heard of curds and whey, now you know what it refers to. When we talk about whey protein, we're usually talking about the powder you'll find in pharmacies, supermarkets and on about a thousand different websites.

Whey protein powder is just a convenient way to take in more protein. It's easily digestible, relatively inexpensive (you can get it for less than 35 cents per 30 g serving if you buy in bulk, which is cheap) and convenient for most people.

It probably goes without saying, but if you're following a decent diet plan, you likely have a daily protein target (somewhere in the range of 2–2.5 g per kg of bodyweight), which you'll want to hit to ensure optimal progress towards your goals. If it's 11pm and you haven't hit your protein target for the day, you could:

- Try to choke down another reheated chicken breast
- Down 2 litres of milk in one sitting
- Take the sensible option and make a nice, filling, easy-to-consume protein shake

You can include whey protein powder in a delicious breakfast smoothie, take it straight with some water, or even use it to replace flour when you're baking (which is a bit tricky, but can be interesting).

There are a number of different types of whey protein: concentrate, isolate, hydrolysed and more. Unless you happen to be lactose intolerant or suffer from digestive issues, you're probably better off sticking with concentrate as it's the cheapest, but the others are worth exploring if you have any special dietary needs. There are also a whole host of non-dairy-based protein powders available on the market. These are mainly for vegans, but they may also appeal to people with whey/lactose intolerances. I've heard the flavour and mixability of these non-dairy powders can be much worse than standard whey, so choose carefully before buying something you won't be able to stomach.

Zinc

Zinc is one of the twenty-four micros essential to your survival, playing a crucial role in the function of enzymes, hormones and your immune system. Zinc naturally occurs in meat, eggs, shellfish (oysters in particular) and legumes. It also acts as a testosterone booster if you're deficient in it (and it goes without saying that more testosterone is good for your progress). If you train hard and you don't get a lot of zinc in your diet, then it's quite possible you're deficient. Zinc is prescribed in the treatment of a number of different health issues, but one of the most widespread uses is as part of a zinc monomethionine aspartate (zma) supplement (which we'll discuss in the next section).

Zinc is readily available in capsule form. It's cheap to take – you can get ninety days' worth of zinc for under €10. Typical (non-prescribed) doses are between 5–15 mg per day, with higher doses of 30–45 mg when you're at risk of zinc deficiency. There are some health risks associated with taking the higher dose for extended periods without good reason, so consult with your doctor if you're not sure. Otherwise, stick with the regular low dose offered in a standard serving of most capsules – it should do you just fine.

Strangely, your body is able to absorb zinc better if you take it along with some green tea. This is down to the unique properties of green tea catechins. If you already drink green tea, consider tying your zinc supplementation to it, but don't worry too much about it. It's not the end of the world if you take it some other time of the day.

You lose zinc through sweating, so if you're training hard and not supplementing with zinc, you're putting yourself at risk of a deficiency. Make the small investment in a decent zinc supplement, take it daily and reap the benefits.

Magnesium

Magnesium is another essential micro. Additionally, magnesium is present throughout your body as an electrolyte (a molecule that supports optimal health and function). Magnesium naturally occurs in foods such as high-quality grains, nuts and leafy vegetables. As these foods are often missing from people's diets, magnesium deficiency is common.

Magnesium has a whole host of functions, and a deficiency causes a lot of health complications, including increased blood pressure, increased chance of depression and declines in cognitive function. It hasn't been shown to have positive effects on exercise performance or body composition, but given the other health benefits it offers you, it's still worth taking.

Magnesium is readily available in capsule form, but it isn't always so easy to find as a standalone; it's often bundled with calcium or zinc. When combined with zinc, it's known as ZMA.

Magnesium comes in a number of different forms. The best one to take is magnesium citrate – it's the most easily absorbed, widely available and relatively inexpensive.

Standard doses of magnesium generally fall in the range of 200–400 mg, depending on your needs. People commonly experience side effects such as diarrhoea and bloating when supplementing with magnesium. To combat this:

• Take your magnesium with food

• Make sure it's mixed well (if it's powdered)

• Reduce the dosage you're taking until you adjust to it

A lot of people take a ZMA supplement to improve their sleep. Having optimal magnesium levels is also associated with improved insulin sensitivity, which has knock-on effects on your physique and health in general.

Supplementing magnesium won't give you super-human strength overnight, but it will support you in pushing hard and progressing towards your fitness goals. As it's fairly inexpensive, I recommend adding it to your regime and seeing how it suits you. The benefits are worth the small cost.

Multivitamins

Multivitamins are one of the most common supplements on the market. There's a good chance you've taken them in the past – maybe you even have some sitting on your shelf right now.

As the name suggests, multivitamins are supplements that contain a number of essential and non-essential vitamins and minerals. There are twenty-four vitamins and minerals that are essential for your survival. Without them, you'll suffer from persistent health problems and suboptimal performance. In an ideal world, you'd get everything you needed from whole foods, but let's be honest here – most of us aren't living exactly like we should 100% of the time. If your diet isn't as perfect as it could be, there's a good chance that you're taking in less of some vitamin or mineral than you should. This can result in you having a subclinical deficiency – not enough to pose a major health risk, but enough to cause problems.

Taking a multivitamin is an insurance policy. It helps you to make sure you're getting enough of what you need (even if your diet doesn't always accommodate this).

Multivitamins come in all forms – regular capsules, powders, effervescent tablets, chewable gummies, liquid. Whatever you're looking for, you'll find it. But as you're going to be taking multivitamins mainly as an insurance policy, you don't need to worry too much about when you take them, or what form you take them in. More importantly, look at what actually goes into the supplement you choose. As a man, the number one thing to avoid is taking a multivitamin with iron in it.

Men have no way of naturally regulating their iron levels, so unless you're anaemic (in which case, consult your GP), you shouldn't be taking in extra iron. A diet rich in lean red meats, chicken and fish will give you all the iron you need.

When it comes to everything else, make sure you choose a decent supplement that covers your bases: multiple vitamins, a relatively high dosage of each (100% of your recommended daily amount or more – google if you're unsure), no iron and at a low cost. Look for these qualities and you'll do just fine. Shop around for the best quality and price. Capsules are dirt-cheap, everything else is a little more expensive (but still manageable).

Taking a multivitamin probably won't change your life, but it will help you in case you're not getting enough of something essential. Considering the low cost and big potential upside, it makes good sense to add a multivitamin to your daily routine.

Fish oils

Fish oil is a common label applied to the two main types of omega-3 fatty acids – eicosapentaenoic acid (EPA) and docosahexaenoic acid (DHA). They're known as fish oils because they're commonly found in fish and seafood in general. These fatty acids can also be found in other foods, but they're cheapest and easiest to get via fish oils.

For health reasons, it's important to keep the ratio of omega-3 to omega-6 acids in your body roughly equal (one to one). As omega-6 acids are abundant in foods like meat and eggs, most people will typically have a suboptimal omega-3 to omega-6 ratio. Unless you're ready to start eating a lot of fish to compensate, supplementing with fish oil is the sensible option.

Fish oil has many health benefits. For starters, taking supplemental fish oil has been shown to decrease your risk of getting different types of cancer or suffering from a heart attack (due to its positive impact on your blood vessels), and it improves bad cholesterol levels in most people.[1] More specifically, fish oil is tremendous for bone and joint health. If you're training hard and putting stress on your body, regularly taking a fish

---

1   I M Berquin, I J Edwards and Y Q Chen (2008) 'Multi-targeted therapy of cancer by omega-3 fatty acids', *Cancer Letters* 269:2, 363, https://doi.org/10.1016/j.canlet.2008.03.044

oil supplement will help to stave off aches and pains, allowing you to push harder in your next session.

Taking fish oil has also been shown to decrease feelings of depression in majorly depressed persons – as much as prescription medication, in some cases. Going along with that, many studies have shown that people who take fish oil experience improvements in mood, general wellbeing, and decreases in anxiety/stress levels.[2] If it's good for the body and mind, there's no reason not to take it – get on it!

Fish oil comes in two primary forms: liquid and capsule. Most people will find the capsules easier to take, so I'd recommend you forget about the liquid (unless you happen to enjoy the taste of cod liver oil). You can (and maybe even should) take as much fish oil as you like without experiencing negative side effects. Start off by taking 1 g per day, gradually scale up until the typical side effects (diarrhoea, nausea etc) kick in, then back off by a capsule or two. To avoid issues with ingesting the capsules, spread your intake throughout the day as you increase the dosages. It's also a good idea to take it with food to minimise any problems.

Fish oil is readily available everywhere. Find one that offers good value for your money, stick with it and reap the benefits over the following weeks and months. With

---

2   www.health.harvard.edu/blog/omega-3-fatty-acids-for-mood
     -disorders-2018080314414

the wide variety of health benefits offered by fish oil, there are few good reasons not to take it.

Steroids

Let me start with a disclaimer: I have never used steroids, and have no plans to use them in the future. I've chosen to write about this topic because I'm often asked about them by young men at the gym – both lads I've worked with and those I only know casually.

As I'm a physical transformation coach, it's my job to know how steroids work, so when someone asks me about them, I can give them an informed answer. One that teaches them about the physical and mental side effects of using these drugs.

First and foremost, I believe that no beginner should ever take steroids while they're new to the gym. To be honest, this is one of the stupidest decisions anyone could make as a lifter (in my humble opinion).

If you want to make the most of powerful anabolic steroids, you need to build a solid foundation first. Without learning to train and eat properly, you'll be shooting yourself in the foot in the long term. This is also likely to happen if you start taking these drugs at a young age, simply because you won't have had enough time to build your foundation. If you lack a deep understanding of how your body works, how to recover from intense training and how to maintain good technique (the kind that targets the right muscle groups and helps you to avoid injury), you'll be wasting your time using steroids. If you don't experiment with bulking and cutting, and learn how your body best responds to fluctuations in volume, intensity and various levels of caloric intake, you'll be wasting your time.

Believe me, all the lessons you learn during years of training as a natural will serve you well if you choose to take steroids later in your career. Get on gear too early, and all you're doing is slapping a band-aid over the gaping wound of your ignorance. But often young men are tempted to take these substances because they lack the patience to learn the valuable lessons that honest, intelligent training as a natural could teach them.

Patience is one of the most crucial virtues you need to succeed as a natural, non-steroid-based lifter (or even an enhanced, steroid-based one, depending on how high you're aiming). If you're not able to delay gratification and put in the work, day after day, you're not going to get very far.

The pros and cons of steroids

When you're on steroids, you make gains much more easily. Regardless of how little you know about effective training or managing recovery, you're practically guaranteed to see results faster than the average natural trainee. And because these gains come so easily, you never have to learn from your mistakes. When everything works, what point is there in learning?

This path of least resistance is actually hugely detrimental to your progress in the long term. And that's assuming you continue to take steroids for your entire life. Here's the thing – the guy who takes steroids early on in his lifting career will often burn out far more quickly than the natural trainee who takes longer to get the same results, but persists along the way.

The reality is that most people who take a few cycles of steroids won't continue to use them for their entire lives. There are a variety of reasons why you might decide to come off them. Maybe your partner objects to them. Maybe the cost gets to be too much. Maybe you need to do it for the good of your health, or you're afraid of getting caught, or you want to start a family. Whatever the case may be, you need to be aware that you won't keep all the muscle you gained while using steroids when you come off them. In fact, you'll lose most of the gains, regardless of how hard you train. And if you're working your arse off and losing most of your gains anyway, what's your incentive to continue? This negative attitude is only exacerbated by your lack of true training knowledge – the kind you would have built if you had taken your time to train as a natural first. With no reason to continue, you'll quit. And then you'll be left with the baggage of potential side effects arising from your steroid usage, with no benefits to offset them.

After you've been training for a good length of time (say five years or more of real, dedicated work in the gym), then you can start to think about steroids if you want to. But before you make that decision, you have to be fully aware of all the ramifications of your choice. Know what you're getting yourself into. You're not just going to experience some mood swings in exchange for getting huge in no time flat – steroids can have a serious and long-lasting impact on your health.

The side effects of steroids

The side effects of using steroids are well documented. Sure, you put on muscle faster and recover from your workouts better than a natural lifter, but the price of those easy gains can take the form of:

- High blood pressure
- Mood swings
- Acne
- Sleep apnoea/difficulty sleeping in general
- Hair loss
- Liver disease
- Kidney disease
- Heart disease
- Testicular shrinkage
- Fertility problems

STRONGER MIND, STRONGER BODY, STRONGER LIFE

None of these side effects are guaranteed, but it's important to be aware of what could happen.

Also, think of what will happen if you come off steroids. Odds are that you'll lose most of the mass you built while using them. Will you be able to cope with not being the big guy in the room? Will you be happy being someone who's just in good shape? Only you can answer that question for sure, but in my experience, people have a hard time re-adjusting when they come off steroids.

Anabolic steroids are a powerful weapon in your training arsenal. But you don't want to use a hand grenade to clean out the spare room when a little elbow grease would do the trick. Think carefully before using them; take them too early and you'll hamstring yourself in the long term.

CASE STUDY: FROM STEROID-FUELLED STRENGTH TO SUSTAINABLE SUCCESS

There were no two ways about it – Bobby was a big man. Tipping the scales at an easy 115 kg, Bobby was the biggest, strongest guy in pretty much any room he walked into. He wouldn't dazzle you with his six-pack, but you could tell he was a serious lifter.

Bobby was a promising rugby player in his youth, but his dreams of lining out as a tighthead prop for the Irish national team took a left turn when he suffered a career-ending knee injury during a routine college game. Without a sport to devote himself to, Bobby had plenty of time to throw himself fully into the process of getting even bigger and stronger than he already was. He added more weight to the bar, added more meals to his regime, tried every supplement under the sun, but eventually, he hit the wall. The gains weren't coming as easily anymore and he was starting to burn out in the gym. Once enjoyable sessions were now little more than a painful distraction.

Bobby could see that he needed to do something drastic to kick start his progression again. And like so many men before him, he decided the best option for getting back on track was to take steroids.

He had never touched them during his rugby career, so when he started to use them as a recreational lifter, the gains were quick and impressive. His lifts moved in the right direction. New muscle stacked onto his already strong physique. And his fire had returned: he was back in the gym five days a week and having a blast. Bobby was repping almost 140 kg on his peak deadlift. He briefly considered training for a national strongman event, but eventually wrote it off as too much of a risk to his knee.

By the time he reached his early thirties, things were starting to change for Bobby. His priorities had shifted. Now a father to twins, he spent his days looking after them and fitting in quality time with his wife whenever he could. He was cycling on and off his steroids throughout this whole time. He was careful – he knew how to manage his doses and avoided most of the nasty side effects that so many others ended up experiencing, but despite his best efforts, some issues arose:

- His moods weren't as stable as they used to be
- His blood pressure was higher than it had been in the past, prompting a visit to his doctor to ensure there wasn't something more sinister at work
- He was starting to feel stiff and immobile when playing with his daughters

Years of pushing the envelope in the gym had put serious stress on his body and the injuries were piling up. Dragging his 115 kg frame around the front garden was tougher than it should have been. Simply put – something had to give. He just didn't know what.

When he came to me, Bobby needed help, but it wasn't going to be an easy process. The main issue was that Bobby had serious mental hang-ups around not being the big guy anymore. He was afraid that coming off steroids for good would leave him small and weak – the complete opposite of the image he'd worked so hard to build.

That's where I came in. Bobby didn't need to be educated about the mechanics of proper training, nutrition and recovery. He already had a solid foundation from his years of natural progression, but I refreshed him on some of the finer details.

We got him on a simple, flexible eating plan, recognising that he didn't need to eat quite as much anymore. We set reasonable weight loss targets that he could easily work towards, helping him to get closer to his (lower) ideal weight. We shifted his training from a five-times-a-week high-intensity routine to a more focused minimalist three-day routine (which fitted better with his busy schedule). Finally, in collaboration with his GP and endocrinologist, we devised a safe – and effective – protocol for getting him off the high doses of steroids he had been taking.

Where is Bobby now? He's not quite as big as he used to be. Rather than lumbering around at 115 kg, Bobby is down to a lean (and much more sustainable) 86 kg. And he's feeling great at that weight. Old nagging injuries don't cause him as much pain and he has tons of energy to play with his kids. His moods are more stable now. Training is something that he does for his health and fitness, but it doesn't define him anymore.

12
Recovery Is Everything

Recovery is the least sexy, but most impactful part of the training equation. Lots of people love pushing themselves hard in the gym. Plenty more enjoy the discipline of sticking to a diet that brings them closer to their goals. But it's rare to find someone who prioritises getting enough sleep.

It's easy to see why. We live in a culture where hustle and grit is glorified above all else. Whether we realise it or not, many of us hold bullshit beliefs about sleep. You've probably heard something like the following before:

- Sleep is for the weak

- Sleep when you're dead

- You have to work harder than anyone else to get ahead, so you can't afford to sleep

These may seem silly when they're written down, but as is the case with most bullshit, there's a small grain of truth to them, and that's what makes them so damaging. If we see successful people doing something, it's natural to think that thing is responsible for their success.

Sometimes, those links are valid. For instance, let's consider a guy who's in great shape. When looking at a stranger like this, we could make different assumptions as to the driver of his success.

1. We could conclude that his consistency and discipline are responsible for his gains

2. We could conclude he has excellent genes and would succeed on any kind of program (not that common, but a possibility)

3. We could assume he takes a particular testosterone booster, or lifts weights in a particular manner, or something else relatively inconsequential

It's the same with sleep. When we see successful people, we may think that their routines or particular habits (the ones they claim to follow, at least) are responsible for their success. So if Hustler x says he only sleeps three hours a night, we can falsely conclude his lack of sleep is the key to his success (while failing to observe his drug habit, industry connections, overwhelming natural talent or anything else).

Getting enough sleep (and managing your stress levels in general) is massively important. It's important if you hope to make progress in the gym, perform your best at work or just be happy in general. If you're consistently sleep-deprived (ie getting less sleep than you'd get if you woke up naturally, without an alarm), then your health, performance and happiness all take a significant hit. You won't have the energy you need to keep moving forward on the path of the strong, and the chances of ultimate failure will skyrocket.

In this chapter, we'll examine the importance of sleep to each area of your life.

Sleep and physical performance

Getting proper sleep is essential if you hope to make real progress in the gym. That's true for a few different reasons.

Anyone who has had trouble sleeping knows that a few days in a row of poor sleep can zap your desire to hit the gym completely. But it's not just your motivation and energy levels that take a hit – it's your endocrine system too. In case you're unaware, let's take a second to talk about why hormones are so critical to improving your health and fitness.

Your body needs certain quantities of different hormones to build muscle, burn fat and improve your fitness. Your endocrine system is responsible for creating all the hormones floating through your bloodstream. You've likely heard many of their names before: testosterone, insulin, oestrogen, leptin, cortisol... the list goes on.

Regardless of their particular name and function, they all serve a purpose. Broadly speaking, your body is constantly fluxing between states of anabolism and catabolism. For the sake of this explanation, think of anabolism as your build-up mode and catabolism as breakdown mode. Depending on the mode you're in, the levels of various hormones your body is using will vary. For instance, cortisol spikes when you're deep in a catabolic state, whereas insulin takes centre stage when anabolism rolls around.

You might think that the goal when you're building muscle is to avoid catabolism entirely and spend all your time in an anabolic state, but that's inaccurate. Catabolism *isn't* always a bad thing. For instance, your body shifts into a catabolic state first thing in the morning to get you going. It does the same when you're working out as it draws on your energy stores to push for more reps, run another lap or bust out one more set.

On the other hand, your body is in an anabolic state when you're resting after a workout, digesting a big meal and yes – when you're sleeping after a long day.

I like to think of catabolism like digging a hole and anabolism as filling it back in. The more digging you do during the day, the deeper the hole gets. The deeper the hole is, the more energy it will require to fill it in.

Maintaining balance between these two opposing states is key. The more time you spend in a catabolic state, the less time you'll have to build muscle and recover from your workouts. And by default, you're either in a state of catabolism or anabolism. That's why chronic stress is so dangerous: it limits your recovery over the course of months and years, which has terrible consequences for your health. So not getting sufficient sleep has a tremendous negative impact on your hormones (specifically the ones that you use to promote muscle growth and strength development).

If you can cast your mind back to the section on training, I cited muscle protein synthesis as an important factor in effective training. Studies have shown that sleep deprivation has negative effects on both your testosterone and insulin-like growth factor (IGF) 1 levels (a precursor to growth hormone production).[1] As

---

1   K A Cote, C M McCormick et al (2013) 'Sleep deprivation lowers reactive aggression and testosterone in men', *Biological Psychology* 92:2, 249, https://doi.org/10.1016/j.biopsycho.2012.09.011

both of these substances are used to promote muscle protein synthesis, having less of them available has obvious consequences for your gains.

Another study compared two groups of people – one sleeping eight-and-a-half hours per night, the other sleeping for five-and-a-half hours.[2] Both groups were placed on a calorie-restricted diet so that they would lose weight. But what kind of weight did they lose?

The group sleeping five-and-a-half hours per night lost 40% more muscle and 60% less fat than the group sleeping eight-and-a-half hours per night. Additionally, the group sleeping five-and-a-half hours per night had higher levels of ghrelin (the hunger hormone) and reported feeling hungrier throughout the day than the other group.

As well as being bad for promoting anabolism, sleep deprivation actively promotes catabolism. Without a chance to recover, your body produces greater levels of stress hormones like cortisol. Higher (temporary) levels of cortisol are a natural side effect of training hard, but are not so great when they arise from your lifestyle choices.

---

2   A V Nedeltcheva, J M Kilkus et al (2010) 'Insufficient sleep undermines dietary efforts to reduce adiposity', *Ann Intern Med* 153:7, 435, www.ncbi.nlm.nih.gov/pubmed/20921542

Here's a simple principle to sum up the importance of sleep. The less time you spend in an artificially stressed-out state, the more energy you'll have when training time comes around.

Intuitively, this makes sense. A hard week at work or family stresses can sometimes leave us less than prepared for a long session in the gym. And we don't need science to tell us that being sleep-deprived will leave us lacking energy to push ourselves. Here's another simple principle. Proper deep sleep allows us to recover from daily stressors (eg training) and gets our endocrine system onside, promoting muscle growth.

That's the quick rundown on why sleep is important for your physical health and performance. But it's not just a question of doing something because it will help you to get fitter; it's also about keeping your mental edge and giving yourself the best chance possible at managing your mood.

Sleep and your mind

Any fool off the street could tell you that functioning on little sleep makes it hard to concentrate. But just how hard?

Shockingly, driving when you're tired is as bad as doing so when you're drunk. Being awake for nineteen hours could be as bad for your focus as drinking a couple of pints before hopping behind the wheel. And don't think the only impact is on your driving abilities. Across the board, sleep deprivation:

- Forces you to make poor decisions
- Increases the chance you'll take unnecessary risks
- Prevents you from correcting your mistakes
- Makes you more forgetful
- Dampens your creativity
- Dramatically impacts your mood

And the truly scary part is that none of us realise how much sleep deprivation affects us. In all of the studies, participants (on average) believed that sleep deprivation had little or no effect on their performance. From their biased perspective, they failed to see the truth. That's because the cumulative effect of losing just a little sleep over the course of a week doesn't feel particularly dangerous. We've likely all thought the same: an hour here, an hour there – it's all good; we can just catch up at the weekend.

I like to use the old analogy of boiling a frog here. If you take a frog and place it in boiling water, it will jump straight back out. But if you let that frog sit in the nice cool water for a while before starting to heat it, it'll stay there and boil alive.

Every hour of rest we deprive ourselves of adds up. We all have enough sense to know that staying up for thirty to forty hours at a time is bad, but few of us realise that over time, we could be pushing our bodies to a place that's almost as dangerous. Like the frog slowly boiling to death in the nice water bath, we might not realise what's going on until it's too late.

And a final word on the link between sleep and your mood: if you think your emotional state isn't linked to your hormones, you're mistaken. Think back on your own life. How often has something seemed like a catastrophe at 2am, but then felt ten times less stressful in the morning?

If you're interested in living a better life, having more brainpower to tackle your challenges head on, making better gains, being more energetic and sharper than ever before, you need to be sleeping well. And if you're not currently sleeping as well as you could be, then read on to discover the best ways to improve your sleep.

Tips to sleep better

The field of sleep optimisation can get pretty weird. I believe that improving sleep should be a priority for anyone who has trouble with it, but you won't see me engaging in two hours of meditation before stretching out on a bamboo sleeping mat for the night. Sometimes,

STRONGER MIND, STRONGER BODY, STRONGER LIFE

the simplest interventions are best. You'll probably find that the solutions to your problems (if you have any) are pretty easy to implement.

In no particular order, here are my top tips for sleeping better.

Get more sunlight

This is a simple one, but not always easy depending on where you live. Sunlight is hugely important in keeping your circadian rhythm (your body's natural energy cycle) on point.

Before electricity was commonplace, people lived in accordance with the rising and setting of the sun. Over the course of hundreds of thousands of years, our bodies became accustomed to this cycle. And fewer than 200 years' worth of programming isn't enough to override our basic functions – sunlight still has an important role to play in regulating our energy systems.

Being exposed to sunlight in the morning, and then more throughout the day, has been shown to have positive effects on people suffering from insomnia.[3] It's quite likely that it would have beneficial effects even if you get enough sleep. If your lifestyle or location

---

3   L Lack, H Wright et al (2005) 'The Treatment of Early-Morning Awakening Insomnia with 2 Evenings of Bright Light', *Sleep* 28:5, 616, https://doi.org/10.1093/sleep/28.5.616

limits the amount of sun you're exposed to, consider investing in artificial substitutes. Search for daylight bulbs or sunshine lamps to get started.

Limit your night-time light exposure

Our lifestyles have changed dramatically in the past 100 years. With the range of entertainment options we have available to us, we can stay awake long into the night, getting blasted directly with sleep-impairing blue light from electronic devices, including smartphones, televisions and computer monitors.

The problem with this (beyond the fact it wastes our time and energy) is that exposure to light at night tricks your body into thinking it's still daytime. So when you head into bed after spending the past three hours scrolling through your phone and mindlessly watching TV, your body isn't ready to sleep.

There are a few different ways you can minimise your light exposure at night. For one, you can set a time in the evening where you shut off your devices and do something else. Read, take a shower, talk to your loved ones, meditate – do whatever you want as long as it's not screen-based. The type of light emitted by electronic devices (blue spectrum light) is the worst offender for tricking your body into thinking it's daytime, but if you have any particularly bright lights in your house, it could be a good idea to switch those off too.

If you still want to use your devices (or have to for work), then consider investing in a pair of blue light blocking glasses. You'll pick up a decent pair on Amazon for under €20. These are designed to filter out the light that keeps you awake while allowing you to enjoy whatever it is you're doing. They're also handy for helping to avoid eye strain if you spend a lot of time on a computer (which more and more of us do these days).

Alternatively, install an app on whatever device you're using to do the same job. F.lux is popular for desktop, and there are a bunch of Android/iOS apps that do the same thing.

Play around with these suggestions and see if it helps. Cut out your screen time an hour before bed and see if that helps. Consider testing a two-hour period. Find whatever works for you. I think that limiting junk media time can only be a good thing anyway, so there's no harm in giving this a go.

Limit your caffeine intake

Like anyone else, I enjoy a good cup of coffee (or two, or six), but I know that drinking too much of it has a bad effect on my sleep. All the things I love about caffeine – its benefits for focus, energy, productivity etc – are actually drawbacks when I'm trying to get better sleep.

Some studies have shown that consuming caffeine within six hours of bedtime can have negative impacts on your restfulness.[4] You might find that your window of safe consumption is longer or shorter than this (it depends on many individual factors), but the point remains: ingesting a lot of caffeine in the late afternoon/evening is probably not a good idea. Limit your caffeine intake to the earlier part of the day and see if it helps you sleep better.

Don't take naps

While napping is a useful tool when you're sleep-deprived (or when you're trying to squeeze in a little more recovery during a busy period of your life), it's nothing more than a band-aid when it comes to solving serious sleep problems. Getting a little bit of sleep during the day can confuse your body into thinking that a new day is starting. That's why you feel refreshed after a good nap, but it's also why napping is bad for regulating your sleep in general. If you are going to take naps, keep them under thirty minutes. Anything more than that impacts your night-time rest too much to be worth it.

If you have persistent sleep issues and are a regular napper, consider cutting them out for a while. You

---

4   C Drake, T Roehrs et al (2013) 'Caffeine Effects on Sleep Taken 0, 3, or 6 Hours Before Going to Bed', *J Clin Sleep Med* 9:11, 1195, http://dx.doi.org/10.5664/jcsm.3170

might find that sleep comes more easily at night once you're tired enough to fall asleep when your head hits the pillow.

Implement a consistent sleep/wake schedule

Your circadian rhythm runs like a clock. If you get it used to habitually switching on and switching off at regular times on a week-to-week basis, you'll soon find that you get naturally tired when your bedtime is approaching. That's why the first few early mornings after a long holiday are so painful. It's also why heading to bed at a reasonable time in anticipation of an early start the next day rarely helps.

Try regulating your sleep patterns. After several weeks, your natural rhythm will adapt and you'll find that you sleep more deeply, wake more easily and feel better throughout the day.

Exercise regularly (but not too close to bedtime)

Exercising regularly (among all the other benefits it gives you) is great for helping you get better sleep. A hard session will give your body the natural push to recover by sleeping more, but remember that exercising too close to your bedtime could have the opposite effect.

Training is a stimulating activity. While you might feel tired afterwards, it's unlikely you'll be able to sleep properly. This is because pushing yourself hard in the gym spikes your cortisol and other stress hormones – great for setting the stage for growth, but less helpful when it comes to getting a good night's sleep.

As with all these tips, try this out and see how it works for you. Shift around your workout times and see how it affects your sleep and energy levels. You might find that early morning sessions are great for you, or maybe the opposite will be true. You'll learn something about yourself either way, so there's no harm in seeing what happens.

Watch your food and fluid intake

Here's another simple but effective tip. Eating heavy meals too soon before bed can be a problem – some people's sleep is negatively impacted by eating a big meal before bed, while other people can actually fall asleep faster on a full stomach. It comes down to whatever you're used to, but if you have digestive issues, it might be a good idea to avoid eating too much late at night.

As for fluids – it's pretty clear that drinking too much close to bedtime will have you making multiple trips to the bathroom, depriving you of precious time in bed and disrupting your circadian rhythm. I like to stop drinking about a couple of hours before bed. If you find yourself waking in the middle of the night on a regular basis, try doing the same.

Optimise your bedroom environment

The environment you sleep in can have a huge impact on how restful your sleep is. There are several different factors to consider here:

• Noise levels

• Brightness

• Temperature

• Comfort

• Function

If you can hear road noise from your bedroom or there's a lot of ambient noise in the area, consider getting some earplugs to reduce the impact this will have on you. Additionally, consider using a white noise machine to drown out annoying sounds like ticking clocks, dripping taps etc.

Darkness is key to a good night's sleep. Feel free to leave some level of light in the room if you want to be able to get up and move around, but limit how much light you're exposed to while in bed. Make the room as dark as you can.

We all know it's hard to sleep when it gets too hot. If you find yourself having this problem on a regular basis, switch off your heating earlier, leave a window/vent open, use a fan, get cooler bedding – whatever it takes.

For comfort, invest in the highest quality bedding, pillows and mattress you can afford. You spend roughly a third of your life in bed, so it doesn't make sense to skimp in this area. I've always found memory foam mattresses to be great, and memory foam mattress toppers are relatively inexpensive. If you have more money to spend, look into getting a gravity blanket (a type of weighted blanket that's supposed to improve sleep quality).

Finally, keep the bedroom for sleep and sex only. Don't spend hours watching TV from your bed – you'll just confuse your brain. Condition your brain to expect either solitude or a good time when you're in bed, and your sleep will undoubtedly improve.

Relax/meditate before bed

This could be as simple as having a solid pre-bed routine that you engage in every night (eg switch off all electronics, read, journal, sleep). But don't think you have to engage in an entire routine or do specific things to improve your sleep. There are a variety of techniques you can employ for this purpose. For instance:

- Taking a hot shower or bath may put you in the mood to sleep

- Journaling about the day as a way of reflecting on what happened can be good if you find yourself lying awake at night, replaying events from the day in your head

• Meditating

• Visualising

• Showing gratitude for what you have in your life

Personally, I like to reflect on my day. I ask myself questions designed to help me understand and analyse everything that happened – what was good, what was bad, what I'm grateful for, what I can do better going forward. It all helps. Doing this allows me to sleep more easily once I get to bed. There's less shit rattling around in my head and I'm better set to face the next day (and all it contains) once it rolls around. If this idea appeals to you, you can do this out loud, in your head or write it all out – it doesn't really matter.

If you find it difficult to wind down at night, consider implementing some kind of relaxation ritual before bedtime. For the short time you spend on it every night, you'll see big results. In general, it's a good idea to minimise your (bad) stress as much as possible. While you need to put a certain amount of pressure on yourself to grow, there's no reason to be wound up and tense throughout the whole day. Being like this will put you on the fast track to failure if you're not careful.

Sometimes, reducing your stress levels is as simple as a shift in mindset – some of the points I share in the first part of this book will help you with that. Other times, you'll have to make hard decisions about what kinds of stress you want to handle. Maybe a relationship will need to be overhauled (or abandoned entirely). Maybe you need to seriously consider finding a new job or making a major life decision. Your mindset is key, but don't suffer unnecessarily. Make decisions in alignment with your goals. Only choose burdens worth bearing. You'll suffer either way, but at least this way, it will be for something meaningful.

If you're generally stressed out, it can help to talk to a professional about what you're going through. Don't be ashamed of doing this; no one is born with inherent knowledge of how their mind works. As a personal trainer, I have never judged people who come to me with a lack of fitness knowledge. That would be silly – no one knows these things without either experiencing them or studying for themselves. In a similar way, I don't judge anyone who needs help learning more about how their mind works, and you shouldn't either. Especially not yourself.

Conclusion

With my background as a personal trainer, I've come across a great deal of information in my time. From working with clients, studying methods used by other trainers and relentless personal experimentation, I've seen what works and what doesn't. What you've read in the pages of this book is the culmination of all this learning – the pure, unadulterated knowledge you can put to use starting today to develop your mindset, build your body, improve your health and hone these critical tools in your arsenal.

Getting into great shape doesn't have to be complicated. Like most things in life, the majority of your results will come from implementing a handful of time-tested principles. Stuff like training for strength, hitting the gym with good frequency, being mindful of your diet and recovering well between sessions – adhering to these guidelines will help you to make gains sustainably without requiring you to spend countless hours in the gym.

Getting your mind right is key, but without a strong body that serves you on the path, you'll never reach your full potential. But with this asset in your corner, your journey to becoming a stronger man and achieving your mission will be made that much easier.

Read back through the chapters. Get a feel for those things you struggle most with, then put that information into practice. If you're currently between workout programs, be sure to visit www.gavinmeenan.com /program and give the sample program a go. If you're currently using one that works well for you, then stick with that – most of the benefit of any routine comes when you stick with it, so don't change things if you're seeing progress.

When you take care of the fundamentals, everything else in life gets easier. You'll have more energy, more focus and more drive. You'll be better able to cope with the stresses of life. You'll be more confident and have an easier time talking to potential partners as a result. The time you spend exercising, eating healthily and recovering from activity will pay huge dividends, so it's worth taking control of this area.

The modern man needs both a strong mind and a powerful body to see his mission through to completion.

You may not be arming yourself for war, but you're still cultivating the attributes of a warrior – men who are dedicated to seeing their unique mission fulfilled. The path is simple, but not easy. The modern warrior must develop himself and his tools to see it through to the end. He understands that all battles are won and lost in the mind long before they're fought in the flesh. Your mindset sets the tone for everything you do; getting it right is 80% of the process.

Through gaining mastery over your mind, you learn how to view the world, overcome challenges and persist in the face of doubt. You build great habits, stoke the fires of motivation and become a fully developed man. You overcome tragedy and setback in all its forms.

With this crucial asset developed, you can turn your attention to your body. Developing high levels of strength and fitness doesn't have to be painful or complicated. Through relentless dedication to the plan, adherence to a handful of high-impact principles and patience, you build the body you need to make your journey easier. The energy you gain from being strong, fit and vibrant will serve you well in all you do. You'll find it easier to remain strong mentally. Life's challenges will be easier to overcome, even welcomed with open arms as a catalyst for growth.

With the mastery you gain over these two critical assets (mind and body), you are well set to conquer the path of the strong man. But to ensure success, you need to tap into the final piece of the puzzle: your heart.

The strong man finds meaning in his mission, but a mission that serves no one but himself isn't enough to keep him moving forward when life gets too hard to bear. By tapping into the power of his heart, he will be able to keep moving, even when the darkness descends and he can hardly see two steps in front of him.

Whether you build a bond with your partner, raise a family, form deep connections with lifelong friends or seek to leave the world a better place than when you entered it, you'll find meaning in engaging with others. This will make the process of successfully completing your mission that much easier, enjoyable and – most of all – fulfilling.

I encourage you to give yourself some time to digest everything we've covered in this book. Some of the ideas may take a couple of reads to fully sink in. You may find that there's one section in particular that stands out for you above all the others. If that's the case, take the time to go through that section in more detail. If you're drawn back to it, it's probably because you know you need to improve in this area.

I encourage you to start small and make gradual changes. Some of the perspectives you've gained from reading this book can show up in your life immediately (eg a new way of looking at things). Other things will take longer to put into practice, such as building better dietary habits. Whatever the case may be, don't neglect to take the most important step:

The first one.

Yes, it's as simple as that. To change your life, you need to start. To walk the path, you must begin.

The information we've covered in this book is a great base to build your knowledge on. For more, follow your curiosity. Read books on the subjects that have jumped out at you as being the most interesting. Talk to people about the ideas you've encountered. Share them with those you consider could benefit from them. And if you're interested in taking things to the next level? I'd be glad to help you do so.

If you're interested in learning more about how I can support you on your journey, please visit www.gavinmeenan.net for more info. Until then, I wish you all the best. The path is challenging, but the world needs more men like you and me. We're making the world a better place, one life at a time.

Yours in strength and health,

Gavin

Acknowledgements

I'd like to take this chance to offer my thanks to everyone who made writing this book possible.

Firstly, I want to acknowledge the services provided by Joe Gregory and all the team at Rethink Press, who have made this book into what you're reading right now.

Thanks to John Clancy for his assistance and invaluable support in writing the book.

Thanks to my good friend and mentor Phil Graham. You've helped me to consistently improve on my business and life, and for that I'm truly grateful.

To the hundreds of clients I've served over the last six years – thank you as well, because without you, none of this would be possible!

And finally, I'd like to thank my family and small circle of friends for being a constant pillar of support throughout the process.

The Author

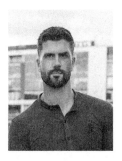

Gavin Meenan is a leading voice in the Irish health and fitness community. A former European Powerlifting Champion, he has personally helped hundreds of people achieve significant physical transformations. Though he's currently based in County Sligo, he works with clients across the world via his online coaching program.

Having reached over 20,000 people with his unique message, Gavin is now expanding his platform into the men's coaching space. His goal is to help men everywhere build stronger minds, bodies and lives.

In his personal life, Gavin overcame struggles such as childhood bullying, trauma, convictions and redun-

dancy. Now, he's on a mission to help other men overcome their challenges too.

For more information, you can follow Gavin Meenan:
🅞 @gavinmeenan
🌐 www.gavinmeenan.net

Printed in Great Britain
by Amazon

67610079R00149